Dermatologic Reactions to Cancer Therapies

Series in Dermatological Treatment

About the Series

Published in association with the *Journal of Dermatological Treatment*, the series in *Dermatological Treatment* keeps readers up to date with the latest clinical therapies to improve problems with the skin, hair, and nails. Each volume in the series is prepared separately and typically focuses on a topical theme. Volumes are published on an occasional basis, depending on the emergence of new developments.

For more information about this series please visit: https://www.crcpress.com/Series-in-Dermatological-Treatment/book-series/CRCSERDERTRE

Dermatologic Reactions to Cancer Therapies

Edited by

Gabriella Fabbrocini, MD
Department of Dermatology, University of Naples Federico II
Naples, Italy

Mario E. Lacouture, MD
Director, Oncodermatology Program
Memorial Sloan Kettering Cancer Center
and
Professor, Department of Dermatology, Cornell Medicine
New York, New York

Antonella Tosti, MD
Fredric Brandt Endowed Professor of Dermatology
Dr. Phillip Frost Department of Dermatology and Cutaneous Surgery
University of Miami Miller School of Medicine
Miami, Florida

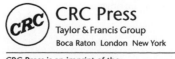

CRC Press
Taylor & Francis Group
Boca Raton London New York

CRC Press is an imprint of the
Taylor & Francis Group, an **informa** business

CRC Press
Taylor & Francis Group
6000 Broken Sound Parkway NW, Suite 300
Boca Raton, FL 33487-2742

© 2019 by Taylor & Francis Group, LLC
CRC Press is an imprint of Taylor & Francis Group, an Informa business

No claim to original U.S. Government works

Printed on acid-free paper

International Standard Book Number-13: 978-1-138-03553-9 (Paperback)
978-1-138-63325-4 (Hardback)

Visit the Taylor & Francis Web site at
http://www.taylorandfrancis.com

and the CRC Press Web site at
http://www.crcpress.com

Contents

v

Contributors

Maria Carmela Annunziata, MD
Department of Clinical Medicine and Surgery
Section of Dermatology
University of Naples Federico II
Naples, Italy

Mackenzie Asel, MD
Department of Dermatology
Northwestern Medical Group
Chicago, Illinois

Mathew R. Birnbaum, MD
Department of Medicine
Division of Dermatology
Albert Einstein College of Medicine
Bronx, New York

Sara Cacciapuoti, MD
Department of Clinical Medicine and Surgery
Section of Dermatology
University of Naples Federico II
Naples, Italy

Mariateresa Cantelli, MD
Department of Dermatology
University of Naples Federico II
Naples, Italy

Gabriella Fabbrocini, MD
Department of Dermatology
University of Naples Federico II
Naples, Italy

Maria Ferrillo, MD
Department of Dermatology
University of Naples Federico II
Naples, Italy

Loren G. Franco, MD
Department of Medicine
Division of Dermatology
Albert Einstein College of Medicine/Montefiore
    Medical Center
Bronx, New York

Azael Freites-Martinez, MD
Department of Medicine
Dermatology Service
Memorial Sloan Kettering Cancer
    Center
New York, New York

and

Hospital Vithas Santa Catalina
Canary Islands, Spain

Peter Arne Gerber, MD, MBA
Department of Dermatology
Heinrich-Heine University
Düsseldorf, Germany

Jae Yeon Jung, MD, PhD
Department of Dermatology
University of Louisville
and
Oncologic Dermatology
Norton Cancer Institute
Louisville, Kentucky

Bernice Y. Kwong, MD
Department of Dermatology
Stanford Health Care
Palo Alto, California

Mario E. Lacouture, MD
Oncodermatology Program
Memorial Sloan Kettering Cancer
    Center
and
Department of Dermatology
Cornell Medicine
New York, New York

Cecilia A. Larocca, MD
Department of Dermatology
Brigham and Women's Hospital/Dana Farber
    Cancer Institute
Harvard Medical School
Boston, Massachusetts

Beth N. McLellan, MD
Department of Medicine
Division of Dermatology
Albert Einstein College of Medicine/Montefiore
    Medical Center
Bronx, New York

Luigia Panariello, MD
Department of Clinical Medicine and
    Surgery
Section of Dermatology
University of Naples Federico II
Naples, Italy

Cataldo Patruno, MD, PhD
Department of Dermatology
University of Catanzaro "Magna Graecia"
Catanzaro, Italy

Tiziana Peduto, MD
Department of Dermatology
University of Naples Federico II
Naples, Italy

Maria Concetta Romano, MD
Dermatology Unit
Ospedale San Camillo
Rome, Italy

Vincent Sibaud, MD
Department of Oncodermatology
Cancer University Institute Toulouse
    Oncopole
Toulouse, France

John David Strickley, BS
School of Medicine
University of Louisville
Louisville, Kentucky

Antonella Tosti, MD
Fredric Brandt Endowed Professor of Dermatology
Dr. Phillip Frost Department of Dermatology and
    Cutaneous Surgery
University of Miami Miller School of Medicine
Miami, Florida

Maria Vastarella, MD
Department of Dermatology
University of Naples Federico II
Naples, Italy

Emmanuelle Vigarios, DDS
Oral Medicine Department
Cancer University Institute Toulouse Oncopole
Toulouse, France

Eric Wong, MD
Department of Medicine
Division of Dermatology
University of Alberta
Edmonton, Alberta, Canada

Jennifer Wu, MD
Department of Dermatology
Chang Gung Memorial Hospital
Linkou, Taiwan

and

Chang Gung University School of Medicine
Taoyuan, Taiwan

1

Introduction to Anticancer Therapies

Jennifer Wu and Mario E. Lacouture

Overview: Cancer Incidence and Types of Systemic Anticancer Therapies

Cancer treatments have revolutionized during the past decades with many new anticancer therapies being developed and approved for a broad variety of cancer types every year (1). More than 10 million people were diagnosed with cancer every year according to World Health Organization (WHO), and 8 million cancer-related deaths and 30 million cancer survivors were reported (2). Accompanied by increased incidence and death, cancer prevention and treatments have become a major issue to public health. Yet the incidences of adverse events to anticancer therapies have also increased in parallel to the rapid emergence of novel treatment modalities, new regimens of combination therapies, and prolonged survival. Different anticancer treatment modalities such as cytotoxic chemotherapy, targeted therapy, immune checkpoint blockade agents, radiation therapy, adoptive T lymphocyte therapy, and hematopoietic stem cell transplantation have distinct spectrums of dermatologic adverse events (AEs), which can involve the skin, hair, nail, and mucous membranes. Dermatologic AEs can not only impair patient's physical function and quality of life but result in dose reduction, regimen modification, and discontinuation of anticancer treatment, which can eventually cause negative impacts on cancer outcomes and even lift-threatening conditions (3). Understanding the epidemiology and clinical manifestations of anticancer therapy–related dermatologic AEs in order to facilitate early recognition, and timely and proper management are important to continue treatments, optimize outcomes, and maintain quality of life. Patient counseling regarding potential dermatologic AEs and strategies for prevention and management before initiation of anticancer therapy is therefore highly recommended. This chapter aims to give a brief introduction on anticancer therapies and their associated dermatologic AEs (Figure 1.1; also see Tables 1.1 and 1.2). The main subjects of each dermatologic manifestation will be discussed in the following chapters.

Anticancer Therapies and Their Associated Dermatologic Adverse Events

Cytotoxic Chemotherapy

Toxic Erythema of Chemotherapy

Toxic erythema of chemotherapy (TEC) describes the overlapping features of skin toxicity induced by chemotherapy through a reproducible nonimmune mediated effect. The clinical characteristics of TEC are erythematous patches or plaques on the axillae and groins, hands, and feet, and, less often, the elbows, knees, and ears, associated with pain, burning, paresthesia, and pruritus. TEC usually appears within days to 3 weeks following the administration of chemotherapeutic agents but may occur late at 2–10 months in patients receiving lower-dose, continuous infusions of 5-fluorouracil (5-FU), or oral agents. Bullae and erosions within the affected area may be seen. The lesions are often self-limited but may recur with readministration of the same agents (4). Hand-foot syndrome (HFS) is a subtype of TEC involving mainly palms and soles (4,5). Chemotherapeutic agents more commonly associated with TEC include cytarabine (AraC), anthracyclines, doxorubicin and pegylated liposomal doxorubicin (PLD), 5-FU, capecitabine

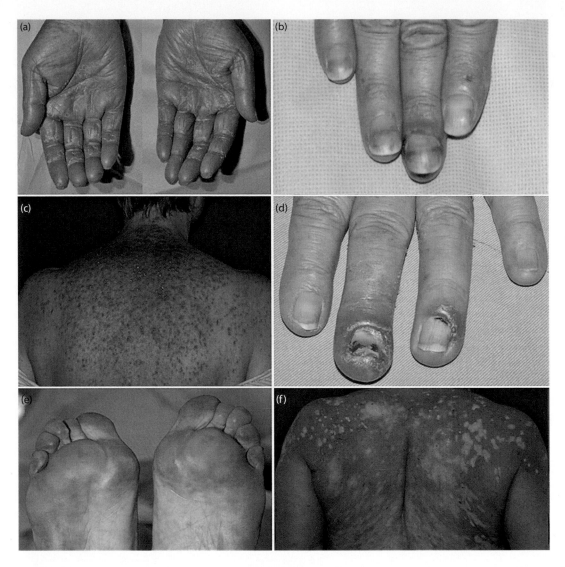

FIGURE 1.1 Dermatologic adverse events to anticancer therapies. (a) Hand-foot syndrome induced by capecitabine (b) swelling of fingertips, subungual hemorrhage, and onycholysis related to docetaxel. (c) Papulopustular eruption related to EGFRI. (d) Paronychia related to EGFRI. (e) Hand-foot skin reaction related to MKI. (f) Vitiligo-like lesions induced by ICIs.

(5-FU prodrug), taxanes (docetaxel and paclitaxel), and methotrexate. Bleomycin, busulfan, carmustine, lomustine, cisplatin, carboplatin, clofarabine, cyclophosphamide, ifosfamide, etoposide, gemcitabine, hydroxyurea, melphalan, 6-mercaptopurine, mitoxantrone, tyrosine kinase inhibitors (imatinib, sunitinib), tegafur, thiotepa, and vinorelbine have also been related to TEC.

Hand-Foot Syndrome

Hand-foot syndrome (HFS), previously named palmar-plantar erythrodysesthesia, is a well-described dermatologic AE induced by certain chemotherapeutic agents (4,5), most commonly capecitabine, 5-FU cytarabine, taxanes, doxorubicin, and PLD (6–10). HFS manifests as dysesthesia and subsequently symmetrical painful erythema and edema of palms and soles. The lesions may progress to blisters, crusts, or ulcerations (10,11). The pathophysiology is not fully understood but believed to be associated with the

TABLE 1.1

Summary of Anticancer Therapies and Their Associated Dermatologic Adverse Events

Types of Systemic Anticancer Therapies	Dermatologic Adverse Events	Common Culprits (Incidence %)
	Hand-foot syndrome (HFS) (palmar-plantar erythrodysesthesia)	Capecitabine (43–63%), continuously infused 5-fluorouracil, cytarabine, docetaxel (5–10%), doxorubicin, and pegylated liposomal doxorubicin (PLD) (45%)
	Immediate hypersensitivity reactions (IHSRs)	Taxanes (30% if without premedication); platinum-based regimens (12–24%) (21)
	Extravasation reactions	Irritants: Platinum-based alkylating agents, taxanes, and topoisomerase inhibitors Vesicants: Anthracyclines, vinca alkaloids, and nitrogen mustards; incidence: 0.1–6% (17,22)
	Pigmentary changes	Busulfan, cyclophosphamide, ifosfamide, bleomycin, 5-FU, vinorelbine, fotemustine, docetaxel, etc.
	Onychodystrophy	Beau's lines: Bleomycin, cisplatin, docetaxel, doxorubicin, melphalan, and vincristine. Onycholysis: Mitoxantrone, docetaxel, anthracyclines, and paclitaxel
	Chemotherapy-induced alopecia (CIA)	
	Chemotherapy-induced acute reversible alopecia	Taxanes are one of the top CIA-inducing drugs (33,34)
	Chemotherapy-induced persistent alopecia (CIPAL)	Busulfan, thiotepa, fluorouracil/epirubicin/cyclophosphamide (FEC) and taxanes
	Radiation recall	Doxorubicin, taxanes, 5-FU, gemcitabine and capecitabine were most commonly reported (44)
EGFR inhibitors (EGFRIs)	Papulopustular eruption (PPE) or acneiform eruption	EGFR inhibitors are used to treat advanced or metastatic non-small cell lung cancer (afatinib, erlotinib, gefitinib, necitumumab), pancreatic cancer (erlotinib), breast cancer (lapatinib, neratinib), colon cancer (cetuximab, panitumumab), head and neck cancer (cetuximab), and in even broader clinical settings based on individual mutations of the tumor (23,49,54)
	Pigmentary changes	
	Changes in hair texture, nonscarring and scarring alopecia, facial hypertrichosis, and eyelash trichomegaly	
	Paronychia	
	Nasal vestibulitis (NV)	
Multitargeted kinase inhibitors (MKIs)	Hand-foot skin reaction (FHSR)	Sorafenib (Nexavar), and sunitinib (Sutent) (9–62% patients exposed to sorafenib and sunitinib, regorafenib, axitinib, pazopanib
BRAF inhibitors (BRAFIs)	Nonmalignant hyperkeratotic skin eruptions	Vemurafenib and dabrafenib
	Cutaneous squamous cell carcinomas (SCCs)	
	Photosensitivity	
	Maculopapular rash (MPR), papulopustular eruption (PPE), or folliculocentric rashes with or without pruritus (53), keratosis pilaris (KP)–like skin eruption on the proximal limbs, trunk, and face (5–9%) (79), and HFSR (80)	
MEK inhibitors		Trametinib, cobimetinib
BRAF inhibitors plus MEK inhibitors		

(Continued)

TABLE 1.1 (*Continued*)

Summary of Anticancer Therapies and Their Associated Dermatologic Adverse Events

Types of Systemic Anticancer Therapies	Dermatologic Adverse Events	Common Culprits (Incidence %)
Hedgehog inhibitors	Alopecia, follicular dermatitis, hypersensitivity reaction, KAs and cutaneous SCCs	Vismodegib, sonidegib
Immune checkpoint inhibitors	Rash, pruritus, vitiligo	Immune checkpoints inhibitors: Anti-CTLA4, anti-PD1, anti-PD-L1
	Autoimmune bullous dermatosis	Anti-PD1 and anti-PD-L1
	Severe cutaneous adverse reactions (SCARs)	Anti-CTLA4, anti-PD1 and anti-PD-L1
Chimeric antigen receptor modified T lymphocytes (CAR-T cell) therapy	Rash (cytokine releasing syndrome [CRS])	CAR-T cell therapy
Radiation therapy	Radiation dermatitis (RD)	Ionized radiation
Hematopoietic stem cell transplantation (HSCT)	Cutaneous graft-versus-host disease (GVHD)	HSCT
Other cutaneous adverse reactions from cancer treatment	Skin infections associated with anticancer treatment (63)	
	Stevens-Johnson syndrome/toxic epidermal necrolysis (SJS/TEN)	SJS: Bendamustine TEN: Bendamustine, busulfan, chlorambucil, fludarabine, lomustine, and procarbazine (Food and Drug Administration Adverse Event Reporting System [FAERS])

apoptosis of keratinocytes induced by cytotoxic chemotherapeutic agents or accumulation of metabolites, which may be enhanced on palms and soles through the transport of sweat (12–14). The involvement of an inflammatory process mediated by the overexpression of cyclooxygenase 2 (COX-2) was also reported (15). HFS can significantly affect the patient's quality of life, limit daily activities, and often necessitates dose modification or even discontinuation of chemotherapy (16).

Acute Hypersensitivity Reactions

Immediate hypersensitivity reactions (IHSRs) usually occur during or shortly after infusion of the first two cycles of chemotherapy with a rapid onset, within minutes (17). The clinical manifestations vary, including nonspecific maculopapular rash, urticaria, angioedema, flushing, and pruritus, with or without constitutional symptoms and signs such as hypotension, dyspnea, or chills (17,18). IHSRs can present as life-threatening anaphylaxis, which requires clinical precautions.

Taxanes (docetaxel and paclitaxel) are most commonly associated with IHSRs with an incidence of 30%, if without premedication. Taxanes have been approved and frequently prescribed for the treatment of metastatic or locally advanced breast cancer, non-small cell lung cancer, prostate cancer, gastric cancer, head and neck cancer, and ovarian cancers (1,17–19). The underlying mechanism is suggested to be related to a hypersensitivity reaction to the solvent for paclitaxel (Cremophor EL®, castor oil vehicle), whereas the solvent for docetaxel (Tween 80, polyoxyethylene-20-sorbitan monooleate) is less frequently implicated (20). Platinum-based agent-induced IHSRs are also observed in 12–24% of patients (21).

Extravasation Reactions

Extravasation reactions occur in 0.1–6% of patients receiving chemotherapy. The severity varies by the volume, concentration, and type of chemotherapeutic agent. The causative agents include irritants (such as platinum-based alkylating agents, taxanes, and topoisomerase inhibitors) and vesicants (such as anthracyclines, vinca alkaloids, and nitrogen mustards) (17,22). Irritants usually cause milder

TABLE 1.2

CTCAE Grading of Dermatologic Adverse Events Associated with Anticancer Therapies

Adverse Events	Grading				
	1	2	3	4	5
Severity	Mild	Moderate	Severe or medically significant but not immediately life-threatening	Life-threatening consequences	Death
Description	Asymptomatic or mild symptoms; clinical or diagnostic observations only; intervention not indicated	Minimal, local or noninvasive intervention indicated; limiting age-appropriate instrumental ADL[a]	Hospitalization or prolongation of hospitalization indicated; disabling; limiting self-care ADL[b]	Urgent intervention indicated	Death related to AE
Hand-foot syndrome (HFS) (palmar-plantar erythrodysesthesia syndrome): A disorder characterized by redness, marked discomfort, swelling, and tingling in the palms of the hands or the soles of the feet	Minimal skin changes or dermatitis (e.g., erythema, edema, or hyperkeratosis) without pain	Skin changes (e.g., peeling, blisters, bleeding, edema, or hyperkeratosis) with pain; limiting instrumental ADL	Severe skin changes (e.g., peeling, blisters, bleeding, edema, or hyperkeratosis) with pain; limiting self-care ADL		
Rash acneiform (PPE): A disorder characterized by an eruption of papules and pustules, typically appearing in face, scalp, upper chest, and back	Papules and/or pustules covering <10% BSA, which may or may not be associated with symptoms of pruritus or tenderness	Papules and/or pustules covering 10–30% BSA, which may or may not be associated with symptoms of pruritus or tenderness; associated with psychosocial impact; limiting instrumental ADL	Papules and/or pustules covering >30% BSA, which may or may not be associated with symptoms of pruritus or tenderness; limiting self-care ADL; associated with local superinfection with oral antibiotics indicated	Papules and/or pustules covering any % BSA, which may or may not be associated with symptoms of pruritus or tenderness and are associated with extensive superinfection with IV antibiotics indicated; life-threatening consequences	Death
Rash maculopapular: A disorder characterized by the presence of macules (flat) and papules (elevated); also known as morbilliform rash, it is one of the most common cutaneous adverse events, frequently affecting the upper trunk, spreading centripetally and associated with pruritus	Macules/papules covering <10% BSA with or without symptoms (e.g., pruritus, burning, tightness)	Macules/papules covering 10–30% BSA with or without symptoms (e.g., pruritus, burning, tightness); limiting instrumental ADL	Macules/papules covering >30% BSA with or without associated symptoms; limiting self-care ADL		

(Continued)

TABLE 1.2 (*Continued*)

CTCAE Grading of Dermatologic Adverse Events Associated with Anticancer Therapies

Grading and Treatment Algorithms for Dermatologic AEs from Cancer Treatments

Adverse Events	Grading				
	1	2	3	4	5
Pruritus: A disorder characterized by an intense itching sensation	Mild or localized; topical intervention indicated	Intense or widespread; intermittent; skin changes from scratching (e.g., edema, papulation, excoriations, lichenification, oozing/crusts); oral intervention indicated; limiting instrumental ADL	Intense or widespread; constant; limiting self-care ADL or sleep; oral corticosteroid or immunosuppressive therapy indicated		
Dry skin: A disorder characterized by flaky and dull skin; the pores are generally fine; the texture is a papery thin texture	Covering <10% BSA and no associated erythema or pruritus	Covering 10–30% BSA and associated with erythema or pruritus; limiting instrumental ADL	Covering >30% BSA and associated with pruritus; limiting self-care ADL		
Photosensitivity: A disorder characterized by an increase in sensitivity of the skin to light	Painless erythema and erythema covering <10% BSA	Tender erythema covering 10–30% BSA	Erythema covering >30% BSA and erythema with blistering; photosensitivity; oral corticosteroid therapy indicated; pain control indicated (e.g., narcotics or NSAIDs)	Life-threatening consequences; urgent intervention indicated	Death
Alopecia: A disorder characterized by a decrease in density of hair compared to normal for a given individual at a given age and body location	Hair loss of <50% of normal for that individual that is not obvious from a distance but only on close inspection; a different hair style may be required to cover the hair loss but it does not require a wig or hair piece to camouflage	Hair loss of ≥50% normal for that individual that is readily apparent to others; a wig or hair piece is necessary if the patient desires to completely camouflage the hair loss; associated with psychosocial impact			

(*Continued*)

TABLE 1.2 (*Continued*)

CTCAE Grading of Dermatologic Adverse Events Associated with Anticancer Therapies

Grading and Treatment Algorithms for Dermatologic AEs from Cancer Treatments

Adverse Events	Grading 1	2	3	4	5
Hand-foot skin reaction (HFSR): A disorder characterized by redness, marked discomfort, swelling, and tingling in the palms of the hands or the soles of the feet	Minimal skin changes or dermatitis (e.g., erythema, edema, or hyperkeratosis) without pain	Skin changes (e.g., peeling, blisters, bleeding, edema, or hyperkeratosis) with pain; limiting instrumental ADL	Severe skin changes (e.g., peeling, blisters, bleeding, edema, or hyperkeratosis) with pain; limiting self-care ADL	—	—
Radiation dermatitis	Faint erythema or dry desquamation (55)	Moderate to brisk erythema; patchy moist desquamation, mostly confined to skin folds and creases; moderate edema (55)	Moist desquamation other than skin folds and creases; bleeding induced by minor trauma or abrasion (55)	Skin necrosis or ulceration of full thickness dermis; spontaneous bleeding from involved site (55)	

Source: Adapted from the Common Terminology Criteria for Adverse Events (CTCAE) grading scale: https://evs.nci.nih.gov/ftp1/CTCAE/CTCAE_4.03_2010-06-14_QuickReference_5x7.pdf.

Note: A long dash (—) indicates a grade is not available. Not all grades are appropriate for all AEs. Therefore, some AEs are listed with fewer than five options for grade selection. Grade 5 (death) is not appropriate for some AEs, and therefore, is not an option. ADL, activities of daily living. BSA, body surface area.

[a] Instrumental ADL refers to preparing meals, shopping for groceries or clothes, using the telephone, managing money, etc.

[b] Self-care ADL refers to bathing, dressing and undressing, feeding self, using the toilet, taking medications, and not bedridden.

inflammatory reaction with the presentation of erythema, edema, and pain. Vesicants can lead to a more severe effect including blister formation, ulceration, and tissue necrosis (23).

Pigmentary Changes

Alkylating agents such as nitrogen mustards (cyclophosphamide, ifosfamide), alkyl sulfonate (busulfan), and nitrosoureas (fotemustine) are commonly reported to result in mucocutaneous hyperpigmentation. Bleomycin, 5-FU, vinorelbine, and docetaxel are also known to cause hyperpigmentation. These skin conditions usually resolve spontaneously and discontinuation of chemotherapy may not be needed (24). Cyclophosphamide and ifosfamide may cause localized hyperpigmentation of the nails, palms, and soles (25,26), whereas busulfan may induce an Addison-like generalized skin hyperpigmentation. Characteristic flagellate hyperpigmentation occurs in 20% of patients treated with bleomycin (27,28). Serpentine supravenous hyperpigmentation is associated with 5-FU, vinorelbine, fotemustine, and docetaxel (29,30).

Hair and Nail Changes

Nail Toxicities

Overall incidence of skin, nail, and hair side effects to chemotherapeutic agents, including taxanes (46%), PLD (7%), other anthracyclines (19%), topotecan (14%), and other agents (14%), is reported to be 86.8%, and among them 23.1% developed nail changes (6). Cytotoxic chemotherapeutic agents can damage the nail matrix and cause transverse ridges across the nail plate, that is, Beau's lines, which are usually self-limited (31). Onycholysis occurs when the nail bed is involved. Pain, paronychia, granulation tissue growth, nail loss, and secondary bacterial infection with abscess formation may complicate onycholysis which can affect the patient's activities of daily living and quality of life (32). Common nail changes related to chemotherapy also include brittle nails, discoloration, splinter hemorrhage, subungual hematoma, and hyperpigmentation (32).

Chemotherapy-Induced Alopecia

Sixty-five percent of patients receiving chemotherapy are estimated to have chemotherapy-induced alopecia (CIA). CIA has been considered the most traumatic impact of chemotherapy by 47% of female patients (33). Taxanes including docetaxel and paclitaxel and anthracyclines are among the most common CIA-inducing agents (33–36). Risk factors include prolonged treatment, higher doses, or multiple exposures (33,37).

Chemotherapy-Induced Reversible Alopecia

Anagen effluvium is a common cause of chemotherapy-induced acute reversible alopecia and typically occurs after the first 4 treatment cycles (37). Any hair-bearing areas including scalp hair, eyelashes, eyebrows, beard, axillae, pubic, and body hair can be involved. Regrowth of hair may be seen 3–6 months after the completion of chemotherapy; however, one-third of patients may experience a decreased amount of hair regrowth and texture and color changes (35).

Persistent Chemotherapy-Induced Alopecia

Persistent chemotherapy-induced alopecia (pCIA) is used to describe the incomplete or absence of hair regrowth lasting longer than 6 months after the cessation of chemotherapy (34). pCIA usually manifests as diffuse hair loss or hair thinning, which tends to be accentuated in vertex areas with clinical features similar to androgenetic alopecia (35,38–42). Eyelashes, eyebrows, axillae, pubic, and body hair can also be affected (39,40,43). Busulfan, thiotepa, fluorouracil/epirubicin/cyclophosphamide (FEC), and taxanes have been reported to cause pCIA (39,40,42). The incidence of pCIA in patients treated with docetaxel was estimated to be around 2% by Kluger et al. but was believed to be underestimated (39). The pathomechanism of pCIA is unclear. A separation of the matrix cells from the dermal papilla and a direct cytotoxic action of taxanes on hair matrix keratinocytes or hair bulge stem cells has been hypothesized (34,39,40).

Radiation Recall

Radiation recall is an acute inflammatory reaction confined to previously irradiated areas triggered by chemotherapy. Doxorubicin, taxanes, 5-FU, gemcitabine, and capecitabine were most commonly reported to be associated with radiation recall phenomenon (44). The incidences are drug dependent and vary from 1.8% to 11.5% (23,45,46). The latency period for radiation recall ranges from several months to years (45,46). Although the pathogenesis remains unclear, a cytotoxic chemotherapy-induced, memory cell–mediated hypersensitivity reaction may play a role (44,47).

Targeted Anticancer Therapy

Targeted therapies achieve anticancer effects through inhibition of specific signaling pathways that play a central role in tumor growth; these include the epidermal growth factor receptor (EGFR) and the intracellular mitogen-activated protein kinase (MAPK) or RAS-RAF-MEK-MAPK pathway (48,49). The emerging profile of dermatologic AEs to targeted anticancer therapies differs from that of cytotoxic chemotherapy. However, the potential to cause dose reduction, discontinuation of anticancer therapy, and impairment of quality of life remain, and may compromise clinical outcomes (50). Therefore, a comprehensive knowledge of prevention, diagnosis, and management of these dermatologic AEs is of paramount importance. Dermatologic AEs have been well characterized for tyrosine kinase inhibitors (TKIs) targeting the EGFR or vascular endothelial growth factor receptor (VEGFR) pathways with various incidences and severity depending on specific targeted therapies and different doses (23,51–54). Common dermatologic AEs related to targeted therapies include acneiform rash, hand-foot skin reaction, xerosis, pruritus, mucositis, alopecia, skin tumors, pigmentary change, and hair and nail disorders (50).

EGFR Inhibitors

EGFR inhibitors (EGFRIs) have been used in broad clinical settings based on individual mutations of the tumor, including advanced or metastatic non-small cell lung cancer (gefitinib, erlotinib, afatinib, osimertinib, necitumumab), pancreatic cancer (erlotinib), breast cancer (lapatinib, neratinib), colon cancer (cetuximab, panitumumab), and head and neck cancer (cetuximab) (23,49,54). Skin toxicities are the most common EGFRI-related AEs, and can manifest as papulopustular eruption (PPE; acneiform rash), xerosis, pruritus, hair, nail, and periungual abnormalities (23,51,52,55). These dermatologic AEs may be painful and debilitating, and may negatively impact treatment intensity, patients' activities of daily living and quality of life (56).

Papulopustular Eruption or Acneiform Eruption

An acneiform rash is the most common dermatologic AE of EGFRI treatment, affecting up to 90% of patients (55). EGFRIs not only inhibit specific signaling pathways on cancer cells but also interfere with signal transduction in normal tissues such as epidermal keratinocytes, sebaceous glands, hair follicle epithelium, and periungual tissues, leading to dermatologic toxicities (23,51,54).

PPE manifests as acneiform follicular and perifollicular papules and sterile pustules on mainly seborrheic areas (face, scalp, and upper trunk), often associated with xerosis and pruritus or even pain (57,58). Skin eruptions are usually transient, appearing in the first few weeks; however, xerosis, pruritus, postinflammatory erythema or hyperpigmentation may persist even after cessation of treatment (56,59).

The development of skin toxicity to EGFRIs was reported to be associated with a favorable cancer prognosis (60). A meta-analysis showed that the presence of rash is associated with a 60% decrease in mortality and a 55% decrease in risk of disease progression in patients with non-small cell lung cancer (60,61).

Pigmentary Changes

A systematic review showed the overall incidences of targeted therapy-induced pigmentary changes of skin and hair were 17.7% and 21.5%, respectively. EGFRI and imatinib were reported to be the most common culprits (62).

Hair and Nail Changes

Paronychia, that is periungual erythema, swelling, pain, with or without periungual pyogenic granuloma-like lesions can develop 2–3 months after the initiation of EGFRI therapy with an incidence varying with different EGFRIs between 12% and 58% (52,63). The lesion is initially sterile but can become superinfected (23). The hypothesized mechanism is periungual inflammation induced by keratinocyte damage and cytokine dysregulation, an effect that may be aggravated by ingrown nails and local trauma (23). Changes in hair texture and color, nonscarring and scarring alopecia, facial hypertrichosis, and eyelash trichomegaly may be seen.

Mammalian Target of Rapamycin Inhibitors

The phosphatidylinositol 3-kinase (PI3K)-Akt-mammalian target of rapamycin (mTOR) signaling pathway is upregulated in multiple malignancies. Dermatologic AEs to mTOR inhibitors, such as temsirolimus and everolimus, are common and include stomatitis, eruptions, and nail changes, including paronychia. mTOR inhibitor–related stomatitis has been reported in 44% of patients and differs from that associated with chemotherapy by presenting as discrete aphthae on nonkeratinizing epithelium (64). Skin eruptions can be seen in one-third of the patients and usually present a maculopapular or papulopustular rash similar to EGFRI-induced PPE (64), which are thought to be related to the inhibition of the PI3K-Akt-mTOR signaling, one of the downstream effector pathways of the EGFR (50).

Multitargeted Kinase Inhibitors

The multitargeted kinase inhibitors (MKIs) such as imatinib, sorafenib, sunitinib, regorafenib, axitinib, and pazopanib achieve their anticancer effects by interfering with molecular signaling pathways involved in cell growth and angiogenesis (65). Dermatologic AEs are most commonly reported in patients receiving MKIs and share overlapping features due to the commonalities among these targeted signaling pathways (23,66,67).

Hand-Foot Skin Reaction

Hand-foot skin reaction (HFSR) is one of the most common dermatologic AEs occuring in 9–62% of patients receiving MKIs such as sorafenib, sunitinib, regorafenib, axitinib, and pazopanib (48,65,68–75). Symmetrical acral erythema associated with desquamation and fissures, followed by hyperkeratosis (presenting as yellowish painful plaques surrounded by an erythematous/edematous halo on pressure areas of the sole) with occasional blister formation is a characteristic feature of HFSR (68).

The proposed mechanism of HFSR include direct pressure and friction to the palms and soles causing the blistering and capillary endothelial damage; disruption of endothelial healing by inhibition of VEGFR and PDGFR; and direct cytotoxic effect to keratinocytes related to dysregulation of the Fas/FasL signaling pathway (48,65,71).

BRAF Inhibitors

BRAF is a serine–threonine protein kinase functioning in the RAS-RAF-MEK-MAPK signaling pathway that regulates cellular proliferation, differentiation, migration, survival, and apoptosis (48,53,76,77). BRAF is mutated in approximately 40–60% of cutaneous melanomas and one of the most frequently mutated protein kinases found in human cancers including hairy cell leukemia, papillary thyroid, serous ovarian, colorectal, and prostate cancers (64).

Dermatologic AEs are one of the most significant and frequent AEs associated with the use of vemurafenib and dabrafenib, occurring in up to 95% of patients (77,78) with a distinct profile including maculopapular rash, photosensitivity, hyperkeratotic lesions, or skin tumors (53). Paradoxical activation of wild-type BRAF cells or cells that harbor a RAS mutation that potentiates the activity of the MAPK pathway results in subsequent keratinocyte proliferation or tumor formation (53,76,77).

Skin Rashes

Rashes are the most common dermatologic AEs, affecting 64–75% of patients treated with BRAFIs, more commonly with vemurafenib than with dabrafenib. A variety of skin rashes can be seen in patients receiving BRAFIs including maculopapular rash (MPR), papulopustular eruption (PPE), or keratosis pilaris (KP)-like skin eruption on the proximal limbs, trunk, and face (5–9%) (79); folliculocentric rashes with or without pruritus (53), and HFSR (80). The occurrence of skin rashes is often within 2 weeks after initiation of treatment.

Photosensitivity

Photosensitivity is a well-known AE occurring in 30–52% of patients receiving vemurafenib, manifesting as acute-onset erythema, burning, and painful blistering with a predilection to sun-exposed areas (53).

Nonmalignant Hyperkeratotic Skin Eruptions

Squamoproliferative/keratinocytic lesions may affect 60–85% patients receiving BRAFIs. Verrucal keratosis is the most common presentation seen in >60% of patients and usually appears early within weeks in the treatment course (53,76,77). Other lesions include palmar/plantar hyperkeratosis over pressure or friction points (40%), skin papillomas, verruca vulgaris, seborrheic keratoses (SKs), warty dyskeratomas, inflamed actinic keratoses (AKs), and keratoacanthomas (KAs) (53).

Cutaneous Squamous Cell Carcinomas

Cutaneous squamous cell carcinomas (SCCs), usually KA type, presenting as rapid-growing, dome-shaped crateriform nodules on sun-exposed skin areas (4–36%) (53,76,77), usually appear early after initiation of BRAFIs such as vemurafenib, with a median onset of 8 weeks (53).

MEK Inhibitors

Upstream mutations at the level of EGFR, RAS, or BRAF can drive constitutive activation within the RAS-RAF-MEK-MAPK pathway, converging on MEK proteins leading to tumor growth (64). Dermatologic AEs of MEK inhibitors (MEKIs), such as trametinib and cobimetinib, share a similar spectrum with that of EGFRIs, including PPE, xerosis, pruritus, alopecia, paronychia, hyperpigmentation, trichomegaly of eyelashes, changes in hair texture, and hypertrichosis of face. PPE is the most common dermatologic AE of MEKIs occurring in 52–93% of treated patients. Secondary bacterial infection to the affected skin area is not uncommon (77,81).

BRAF Inhibitors plus MEK Inhibitors

Combination therapy of a BRAFI plus a MEKI seems to show an improved skin toxicity profile than a BRAFI alone due to the effect of downstream MEK inhibition on the paradoxical activation of the MAPK pathway by BRAF inhibitors (64). The combination of dabrafenib with trametinib showed a significant decrease of incidence of cutaneous SCCs (0% versus 26.1%), verrucal keratosis, and Grover's disease compared to that of dabrafenib alone, but a higher frequency of folliculitis (40% versus 6.7%) (76,77,82,83).

Hedgehog Pathway Inhibitors (Vismodegib, Sonidegib)

Abnormal activation of hedgehog pathway signaling is a key driver in the pathogenesis of basal cell carcinoma (BCC). Vismodegib and sonidegib, small molecule inhibitors of hedgehog pathway signaling, are approved for the treatment of adults who have metastatic BCC or locally advanced BCC in selected patients. Commonly observed AEs include muscle spasms, ageusia/dysgeusia, alopecia, weight loss, and fatigue (84).

Alopecia is a common dermatologic AE to hedgehog pathway inhibitors affecting 46–66% of treated patients and has a relatively delayed onset than that with cytotoxic chemotherapy, developing after 2 months of treatment (84–87). The mechanism may be related to the important role that the hedgehog pathway plays in the normal hair follicle cycle. Follicle-based toxicities, such as alopecia and folliculitis, are hypothesized to be possible surrogate markers of tumor response (85). Follicular dermatitis, hypersensitivity reaction, KAs, and cutaneous SCCs have also been reported (84–91).

Immune Checkpoint Inhibitors

The cytotoxic T lymphocyte antigen-4 (CTLA-4) signaling pathway, and the programmed cell death receptor-1 (PD-1)/PD ligand-1 (PD-L1) signaling pathway are immune checkpoints of immunologic homeostasis and tumor-induced immune suppression (92). As immune checkpoint inhibitors (ICIs) restore antitumor immunity by interrupting the inhibitory signals and immune escape mechanisms induced by tumor cells, they may concurrently induce autoimmunity and inflammation of various organ systems, most commonly the skin, gastrointestinal tract, endocrine glands, and liver, referred to as immune-related adverse events (irAEs) (93–95).

The precise pathogenesis underlying dermatologic irAEs remains to be elucidated. Possible mechanisms include increasing T-cell activity against common antigens that are presented in both tumors and healthy tissue, for example, vitiligo; increasing levels of preexisting autoantibodies, for example, bullous pemphigoid; and increasing levels of inflammatory cytokines, for example, psoriasis and psoriasiform rash (95).

Pruritus, Rash, and Vitiligo

Immune-related dermatologic AEs are among the earliest and most common AEs of ICIs, which include pruritus, rash, and vitiligo. Vitiligo is more frequently seen in patients with melanoma (94,96–98). Autoimmune bullous dermatoses (99), lichenoid dermatitis/mucositis, exacerbated psoriasis, psoriasiform rash, alopecia areata/universalis, Stevens-Johnson syndrome (SJS), and toxic epidermal necrosis (TEN) have been anecdotally reported (93,98,100–104). Increasing evidence suggest that vitiligo and/or rash developing during ICI treatments are correlated to favorable clinical outcomes (92,103,105–107).

Bullous Pemphigoid

Bullous pemphigoid (BP) may develop in patients receiving an anti-PD1/PD-L1 treatment and is thought to be mediated by both T-cell and B-cell immunity (99,108). BP associated with ICIs may occur accompanied or preceded by pruritus within months after the initiation of ICIs, and may persist after cessation of treatment. Skin biopsy, direct and indirect immunofluorescence study of skin and serum autoantibodies such as anti-BP180 and anti-BP230 may be helpful for diagnosis (99).

Severe Cutaneous Adverse Reactions

Severe cutaneous adverse reactions (SCARs) are rare, but SJS, TEN, and drug reaction with eosinophilia and systemic symptoms (DRESS) syndrome associated with ICIs were reported in the literature (109–111). A comprehensive review of clinical and drug history is necessary for accurate diagnosis and attribution of the culprit.

Chimeric Antigen Receptor-Modified T Lymphocytes Therapy

Adoptive cell therapy is a powerful and promising approach to cancer therapy. Cytokine release syndrome (CRS) can be observed shortly after administration of chimeric antigen receptor-modified T lymphocytes (CAR-T cell) therapy (92). Autoimmunity induced by administered T cells may occur when a T-cell receptor (TCR) targeting a protein is expressed in normal tissue, for example, when proteins of melanocytic origin are targeted with TCRs against melanoma antigen recognized by T cells 1 (MART-1) and glycoprotein 100, cutaneous, ocular, and internal ear toxicities occur (92).

Radiation Therapy

Radiation Dermatitis

Radiation dermatitis often occurs approximately 2–3 weeks after the initiation of radiotherapy (112). Acute radiation dermatitis, usually manifesting as erythema, dry and moist desquamation, and ulceration, is self-limiting and usually resolves after 2–3 months. Late toxicities usually occur later in the treatment course at greater than 90 days. Skin lesions include telangiectasia, atrophy, fibrosis, edema, and ulceration, which may persist and result in a prolonged negative impact on a patient's quality of life (55,112,113).

Hematopoietic Stem Cell Transplantation

Cutaneous Graft-versus-Host Disease

Graft-versus-host disease (GVHD) is a major complication of allogeneic hematopoietic stem cell transplant (allo-HSCT) recipients with an incidence of 40–60%, and accounts for 15% of treatment-related deaths (114,115). Cutaneous GVHD is the most common to appear, affecting 60–80% of patients, which can result in long-term complications such as cosmetic, functional, and even life-threatening sequelae (114,115). Characteristic manifestations of cutaneous GVHD are poikiloderma, lichen planus–like eruptions, lichen sclerosus–like lesions, morphea-like sclerosis, and deep sclerosis or fasciitis (114).

Conclusion

Maintaining patients on an anticancer treatment is critical for cancer survival. The rapid development of novel therapies brings promising anticancer efficacy along with a wide variety of undesirable AEs. Dermatologic AEs are among the most frequently observed and may seriously impair patients' quality of life. Increasing evidence suggests that these dermatologic AEs are preventable and manageable by comprehensive pretreatment counseling, preemptive treatment, early diagnosis, and proper management. Dermatologists play a critical role in minimizing the impact of dermatologic AEs. Early and prompt dermatology referral and a multidiscipline team including dermatologists are beneficial for optimal cancer care.

REFERENCES

1. Giavina-Bianchi P, Patil SU, Banerji A. Immediate hypersensitivity reaction to chemotherapeutic agents. *J Allergy Clin Immunol Pract* 2017;5(3):593–9.
2. Santoni M et al. Risk of pruritus in cancer patients treated with biological therapies: A systematic review and meta-analysis of clinical trials. *Crit Rev Oncol Hematol* 2015;96(2):206–19.
3. Lacouture ME. Management of dermatologic toxicities. *JNCCN* 2015;13(5 Suppl):686–9.
4. Bolognia JL, Cooper DL, Glusac EJ. Toxic erythema of chemotherapy: A useful clinical term. *J Am Acad Dermatol* 2008;59(3):524–9.
5. Parker TL, Cooper DL, Seropian SE, Bolognia JL. Toxic erythema of chemotherapy following i.v. BU plus fludarabine for allogeneic PBSC transplant. *Bone Marrow Transplant* 2013;48(5):646–50.
6. Hackbarth M, Haas N, Fotopoulou C, Lichtenegger W, Sehouli J. Chemotherapy-induced dermatological toxicity: Frequencies and impact on quality of life in women's cancers. Results of a prospective study. *Support Care Cancer* 2008;16(3):267–73.
7. Saif MW, Katirtzoglou NA, Syrigos KN. Capecitabine: An overview of the side effects and their management. *Anti-Cancer Drugs* 2008;19(5):447–64.
8. Chew L, Chuen VS. Cutaneous reaction associated with weekly docetaxel administration. *J Oncol Pharm Pract: ISOPP* 2009;15(1):29–34.
9. Balagula Y, Rosen ST, Lacouture ME. The emergence of supportive oncodermatology: The study of dermatologic adverse events to cancer therapies. *J Am Acad Dermatol* 2011;65(3):624–35.
10. Lorusso D, Di Stefano A, Carone V, Fagotti A, Pisconti S, Scambia G. Pegylated liposomal doxorubicin-related palmar-plantar erythrodysesthesia ('hand-foot' syndrome). *Ann Oncol: ESMO* 2007;18(7):1159–64.
11. von Moos R et al. Pegylated liposomal doxorubicin-associated hand-foot syndrome: Recommendations of an international panel of experts. *Eur J Cancer* 2008;44(6):781–90.
12. Chen M et al. The contribution of keratinocytes in capecitabine-stimulated hand-foot-syndrome. *Environ Toxicol Pharmacol* 2017;49:81–8.
13. Yang J et al. The role of the ATM/Chk/P53 pathway in mediating DNA damage in hand-foot syndrome induced by PLD. *Toxicol Lett* 2017;265:131–9.

14. Lou Y et al. Possible pathways of capecitabine-induced hand-foot syndrome. *Chem Res Toxicol* 2016;29(10):1591–601.
15. Zhang RX et al. Celecoxib can prevent capecitabine-related hand-foot syndrome in stage II and III colorectal cancer patients: Result of a single-center, prospective randomized phase III trial. *Ann Oncol: ESMO* 2012;23(5):1348–53.
16. Nikolaou V, Syrigos K, Saif MW. Incidence and implications of chemotherapy related hand-foot syndrome. *Expert Opin Drug Saf* 2016;15(12):1625–33.
17. Sibaud V, Meyer N, Lamant L, Vigarios E, Mazieres J, Delord JP. Dermatologic complications of anti-PD-1/PD-L1 immune checkpoint antibodies. *Curr Opin Oncol* 2016;28(4):254–63.
18. Syrigou E et al. Hypersensitivity reactions to docetaxel: Retrospective evaluation and development of a desensitization protocol. *Int Arch Allergy Immunol* 2011;156(3):320–4.
19. Aoyama T et al. Is there any predictor for hypersensitivity reactions in gynecologic cancer patients treated with paclitaxel-based therapy? *Cancer Chemother Pharmacol* 2017;80(1):65–9.
20. Gelmon K. The taxoids: Paclitaxel and docetaxel. *Lancet* 1994;344(8932):1267–72.
21. Park HJ et al. A new practical desensitization protocol for oxaliplatin-induced immediate hypersensitivity reactions: A necessary and useful approach. *J Investig Allergol Clin Immunol* 2016;26(3):168–76.
22. Langer SW. Extravasation of chemotherapy. *Curr Oncol Rep* 2010;12(4):242–6.
23. Kyllo R, Anadkat M. Dermatologic adverse events to chemotherapeutic agents, Part 1: Cytotoxic agents, epidermal growth factor inhibitors, multikinase inhibitors, and proteasome inhibitors. *Semin Cutan Med Surg* 2014;33(1):28–39.
24. Jain V, Bhandary S, Prasad GN, Shenoi SD. Serpentine supravenous streaks induced by 5-fluorouracil. *J Am Acad Dermatol* 2005;53(3):529–30.
25. Teresi ME, Murry DJ, Cornelius AS. Ifosfamide-induced hyperpigmentation. *Cancer* 1993;71(9): 2873–5.
26. Chittari K, Tagboto S, Tan BB. Cyclophosphamide-induced nail discoloration and skin hyperpigmentation: A rare presentation. *Clin Exp Dermatol* 2009;34(3):405–6.
27. Abess A, Keel DM, Graham BS. Flagellate hyperpigmentation following intralesional bleomycin treatment of verruca plantaris. *Arch Dermatol* 2003;139(3):337–9.
28. Vuerstaek JD, Frank J, Poblete-Gutierrez P. Bleomycin-induced flagellate dermatitis. *Int J Dermatol* 2007(46 Suppl 3):3–5.
29. Huang V, Anadkat M. Dermatologic manifestations of cytotoxic therapy. *Dermatol Ther* 2011;24(4): 401–10.
30. Suvirya S, Agrawal A, Parihar A. 5-Fluorouracil-induced bilateral persistent serpentine supravenous hyperpigmented eruption, bilateral mottling of palms and diffuse hyperpigmentation of soles. *BMJ Case Reports* 2014;2014.
31. Kyllo RL, Anadkat MJ. Dermatologic adverse events to chemotherapeutic agents, part 1: Cytotoxics, epidermal growth factor receptors, multikinase inhibitors, and proteasome inhibitors. *Semin Cutan Med Surg* 2014;33(1):28–39.
32. Capriotti K et al. The risk of nail changes with taxane chemotherapy: A systematic review of the literature and meta-analysis. *Br J Dermatol* 2015;173(3):842–5.
33. Trueb RM. Chemotherapy-induced hair loss. *Skin Therapy Lett* 2010;15(7):5–7.
34. Tallon B, Blanchard E, Goldberg LJ. Permanent chemotherapy-induced alopecia: Case report and review of the literature. *J Am Acad Dermatol* 2010;63(2):333–6.
35. Lindner J et al. Hair shaft abnormalities after chemotherapy and tamoxifen therapy in patients with breast cancer evaluated by optical coherence tomography. *Br J Dermatol* 2012;167(6):1272–8.
36. Nangia J et al. Effect of a scalp cooling device on alopecia in women undergoing chemotherapy for breast cancer: The SCALP randomized clinical trial. *JAMA* 2017;317(6):596–605.
37. Trueb RM. Chemotherapy-induced anagen effluvium: Diffuse or patterned? *Dermatology* 2007; 215(1):1–2.
38. Fonia A, Cota C, Setterfield JF, Goldberg LJ, Fenton DA, Stefanato CM. Permanent alopecia in patients with breast cancer after taxane chemotherapy and adjuvant hormonal therapy: Clinicopathologic findings in a cohort of 10 patients. *J Am Acad Dermatol* 2017;76(5):948–57.
39. Kluger N et al. Permanent scalp alopecia related to breast cancer chemotherapy by sequential fluorouracil/epirubicin/cyclophosphamide (FEC) and docetaxel: A prospective study of 20 patients. *Ann Oncol: ESMO* 2012;23(11):2879–84.

40. Miteva M, Misciali C, Fanti PA, Vincenzi C, Romanelli P, Tosti A. Permanent alopecia after systemic chemotherapy: A clinicopathological study of 10 cases. *Am J Dermatopathol* 2011;33(4):345–50.
41. Asz-Sigall D, Gonzalez-de-Cossio-Hernandez AC, Rodriguez-Lobato E, Ortega-Springall MF, Vega-Memije ME, Arenas Guzman R. Differential diagnosis of female-pattern hair loss. *Skin Appendage Disord* 2016;2(1–2):18–21.
42. Palamaras I, Misciali C, Vincenzi C, Robles WS, Tosti A. Permanent chemotherapy-induced alopecia: A review. *J Am Acad Dermatol* 2011;64(3):604–6.
43. Prevezas C, Matard B, Pinquier L, Reygagne P. Irreversible and severe alopecia following docetaxel or paclitaxel cytotoxic therapy for breast cancer. *Br J Dermatol* 2009;160(4):883–5.
44. Burris HA, 3rd, Hurtig J. Radiation recall with anticancer agents. *Oncologist* 2010;15(11):1227–37.
45. Sanborn RE, Sauer DA. Cutaneous reactions to chemotherapy: Commonly seen, less described, little understood. *Dermatol Clin* 2008;26(1):103–19, ix.
46. Wyatt AJ, Leonard GD, Sachs DL. Cutaneous reactions to chemotherapy and their management. *Am J Clin Dermatol* 2006;7(1):45–63.
47. Korman AM, Tyler KH, Kaffenberger BH. Radiation recall dermatitis associated with nivolumab for metastatic malignant melanoma. *Int J Dermatol* 2017;56(4):e75–7.
48. Belum VR, Fontanilla Patel H, Lacouture ME, Rodeck U. Skin toxicity of targeted cancer agents: Mechanisms and intervention. *Future Oncol* 2013;9(8):1161–70.
49. Tang N, Ratner D. Managing cutaneous side effects from targeted molecular inhibitors for melanoma and nonmelanoma skin cancer. *Dermatol Surg* 2016;42(Suppl 1):S40–8.
50. Belum VR, Washington C, Pratilas CA, Sibaud V, Boralevi F, Lacouture ME. Dermatologic adverse events in pediatric patients receiving targeted anticancer therapies: A pooled analysis. *Pediatr Blood Cancer* 2015;62(5):798–806.
51. Lacouture ME, Ciccolini K, Kloos RT, Agulnik M. Overview and management of dermatologic events associated with targeted therapies for medullary thyroid cancer. *Thyroid* 2014;24(9):1329–40.
52. Lacouture ME et al. Clinical practice guidelines for the prevention and treatment of EGFR inhibitor-associated dermatologic toxicities. *Support Care Cancer* 2011;19(8):1079–95.
53. Belum VR, Fischer A, Choi JN, Lacouture ME. Dermatological adverse events from BRAF inhibitors: A growing problem. *Curr Oncol Rep* 2013;15(3):249–59.
54. Tischer B, Huber R, Kraemer M, Lacouture ME. Dermatologic events from EGFR inhibitors: The issue of the missing patient voice. *Support Care Cancer* 2017;25(2):651–60.
55. Lacouture ME et al. A proposed EGFR inhibitor dermatologic adverse event-specific grading scale from the MASCC skin toxicity study group. *Support Care Cancer* 2010;18(4):509–22.
56. Hofheinz RD et al. Recommendations for the prophylactic management of skin reactions induced by epidermal growth factor receptor inhibitors in patients with solid tumors. *Oncologist* 2016;21(12):1483–91.
57. Hsiao YW, Lin YC, Hui RC, Yang CH. Fulminant acneiform eruptions after administration of dovitinib in a patient with renal cell carcinoma. *J Clin Oncol* 2011;29(12):e340–1.
58. Drilon A et al. Beyond the dose-limiting toxicity period: Dermatologic adverse events of patients on phase 1 trials of the cancer therapeutics evaluation program. *Cancer* 2016;122(8):1228–37.
59. Clabbers JMK et al. Xerosis and pruritus as major EGFRI-associated adverse events. *Support Care Cancer* 2016;24(2):513–21.
60. Liu HB et al. Skin rash could predict the response to EGFR tyrosine kinase inhibitor and the prognosis for patients with non-small cell lung cancer: A systematic review and meta-analysis. *PLoS One* 2013;8(1):e55128.
61. Lacouture ME et al. Skin toxicity evaluation protocol with panitumumab (STEPP), a phase II, open-label, randomized trial evaluating the impact of a pre-emptive skin treatment regimen on skin toxicities and quality of life in patients with metastatic colorectal cancer. *J Clin Oncol* 2010;28(8):1351–7.
62. Dai J, Belum VR, Wu S, Sibaud V, Lacouture ME. Pigmentary changes in patients treated with targeted anticancer agents: A systematic review and meta-analysis. *J Am Acad Dermatol* 2017;77(5):902–10.e2.
63. Gandhi M, Brieva JC, Lacouture ME. Dermatologic infections in cancer patients. *Cancer Treat Res* 2014;161:299–317.
64. Macdonald JB, Macdonald B, Golitz LE, LoRusso P, Sekulic A. Cutaneous adverse effects of targeted therapies: Part II: Inhibitors of intracellular molecular signaling pathways. *J Am Acad Dermatol* 2015;72(2):221–36, quiz 37–8.
65. Lacouture ME et al. Evolving strategies for the management of hand-foot skin reaction associated with the multitargeted kinase inhibitors sorafenib and sunitinib. *Oncologist* 2008;13(9):1001–11.

66. Valentine J et al. Incidence and risk of xerosis with targeted anticancer therapies. *J Am Acad Dermatol* 2015;72(4):656–67.
67. Ensslin CJ, Rosen AC, Wu S, Lacouture ME. Pruritus in patients treated with targeted cancer therapies: Systematic review and meta-analysis. *J Am Acad Dermatol* 2013;69(5):708–20.
68. Gomez P, Lacouture ME. Clinical presentation and management of hand-foot skin reaction associated with sorafenib in combination with cytotoxic chemotherapy: Experience in breast cancer. *Oncologist* 2011;16(11):1508–19.
69. Lacouture ME, Reilly LM, Gerami P, Guitart J. Hand foot skin reaction in cancer patients treated with the multikinase inhibitors sorafenib and sunitinib. *Ann Oncol: ESMO* 2008;19(11):1955–61.
70. Lacouture ME et al. Dermatologic adverse events associated with afatinib: An oral ErbB family blocker. *Expert Rev Anticancer Ther* 2013;13(6):721–8.
71. Yeh CN et al. Fas/Fas ligand mediates keratinocyte death in sunitinib-induced hand-foot skin reaction. *J Invest Dermatol* 2014;134(11):2768–75.
72. Belum VR, Wu S, Lacouture ME. Risk of hand-foot skin reaction with the novel multikinase inhibitor regorafenib: A meta-analysis. *Investig New Drugs* 2013;31(4):1078–86.
73. Fischer A, Wu S, Ho AL, Lacouture ME. The risk of hand-foot skin reaction to axitinib, a novel VEGF inhibitor: A systematic review of literature and meta-analysis. *Investig New Drugs* 2013;31(3):787–97.
74. McLellan B, Ciardiello F, Lacouture ME, Segaert S, Van Cutsem E. Regorafenib-associated hand-foot skin reaction: Practical advice on diagnosis, prevention, and management. *Ann Oncol: ESMO* 2015;26(10):2017–26.
75. Balagula Y, Wu S, Su X, Feldman DR, Lacouture ME. The risk of hand foot skin reaction to pazopanib, a novel multikinase inhibitor: A systematic review of literature and meta-analysis. *Investig New Drugs* 2012;30(4):1773–81.
76. Carlos G et al. Cutaneous toxic effects of BRAF inhibitors alone and in combination with MEK inhibitors for metastatic melanoma. *JAMA Dermatol* 2015;151(10):1103–9.
77. Choi JN. Dermatologic adverse events to chemotherapeutic agents, Part 2: BRAF inhibitors, MEK inhibitors, and ipilimumab. *Semin Cutan Med Surg* 2014;33(1):40–8.
78. Belum VR, Cercek A, Sanz-Motilva V, Lacouture ME. Dermatologic adverse events to targeted therapies in lower GI cancers: Clinical presentation and management. *Curr Treat Options Oncol* 2013;14(3):389–404.
79. Pugliese SB, Neal JW, Kwong BY. Management of dermatologic complications of lung cancer therapies. *Curr Treat Options Oncol* 2015;16(10):50.
80. Chandrakumar SF, Yeung J. Cutaneous adverse events during vemurafenib therapy. *J Cutan Med Surg* 2014;18(4):223–8.
81. Balagula Y, Barth Huston K, Busam KJ, Lacouture ME, Chapman PB, Myskowski PL. Dermatologic side effects associated with the MEK 1/2 inhibitor selumetinib (AZD6244, ARRY-142886). *Investig New Drugs* 2011;29(5):1114–21.
82. Dreno B et al. Incidence, course, and management of toxicities associated with cobimetinib in combination with vemurafenib in the coBRIM study. *Ann Oncol: ESMO* 2017;28(5):1137–44.
83. Keating GM. Cobimetinib plus vemurafenib: A review in BRAF (V600) mutation-positive unresectable or metastatic melanoma. *Drugs* 2016;76(5):605–15.
84. Lacouture ME et al. Characterization and management of hedgehog pathway inhibitor-related adverse events in patients with advanced basal cell carcinoma. *Oncologist* 2016;21(10):1218–29.
85. Kwong B, Danial C, Liu A, Chun KA, Chang AL. Reversible cutaneous side effects of vismodegib treatment. *Cutis* 2017;99(3):19–20.
86. LoRusso PM et al. Phase I trial of hedgehog pathway inhibitor vismodegib (GDC-0449) in patients with refractory, locally advanced or metastatic solid tumors. *Clin Cancer Res* 2011;17(8):2502–11.
87. Sekulic A et al. Long-term safety and efficacy of vismodegib in patients with advanced basal cell carcinoma: final update of the pivotal ERIVANCE BCC study. *BMC Cancer* 2017;17(1):332.
88. Aasi S et al. New onset of keratoacanthomas after vismodegib treatment for locally advanced basal cell carcinomas: A report of 2 cases. *JAMA Dermatol* 2013;149(2):242–3.
89. Sekulic A et al. Efficacy and safety of vismodegib in advanced basal-cell carcinoma. *N Engl J Med* 2012;366(23):2171–9.
90. U.S. Food and Drug Administration. Vismodegib. January 2012. https://www.accessdata.fda.gov/drugsatfda_docs/label/2012/203388lbl.pdf. Accessed June 26, 2017.

91. European Medicines Agency. European Public Assessment Report: Erivedge. October 2016. http://www.ema.europa.eu/docs/en_GB/document_library/EPAR_-_Summary_for_the_public/human/002602/WC500146821.pdf.

92. Weber JS, Yang JC, Atkins MB, Disis ML. Toxicities of immunotherapy for the practitioner. *J Clin Oncol* 2015;33(18):2092–9.

93. Michot JM et al. Immune-related adverse events with immune checkpoint blockade: A comprehensive review. *Eur J Cancer* 2016;54:139–48.

94. Wolchok JD et al. Ipilimumab monotherapy in patients with pretreated advanced melanoma: A randomised, double-blind, multicentre, phase 2, dose-ranging study. *Lancet Oncol* 2010;11(2):155–64.

95. Postow MA, Sidlow R, Hellmann MD. Immune-related adverse events associated with immune checkpoint blockade. *N Engl J Med* 2018;378(2):158–68.

96. Larsabal M et al. Vitiligo-like lesions occurring in patients receiving anti-programmed cell death-1 therapies are clinically and biologically distinct from vitiligo. *J Am Acad Dermatol* 2017;76(5):863–70.

97. Belum VR et al. Characterisation and management of dermatologic adverse events to agents targeting the PD-1 receptor. *Eur J Cancer* 2016;60:12–25.

98. Robert C et al. Pembrolizumab versus ipilimumab in advanced melanoma. *N Engl J Med* 2015;372(26):2521–32.

99. Naidoo J et al. Autoimmune bullous skin disorders with immune checkpoint inhibitors targeting PD-1 and PD-L1. *Cancer Immunol Res* 2016;4(5):383–9.

100. Damsky W, King BA. JAK inhibitors in dermatology: The promise of a new drug class. *J Am Acad Dermatol* 2017;76(4):736–44.

101. Shreberk-Hassidim R, Ramot Y, Zlotogorski A. Janus kinase inhibitors in dermatology: A systematic review. *J Am Acad Dermatol* 2017;76(4):745–53.e19.

102. Sibaud V et al. Oral lichenoid reactions associated with anti-PD-1/PD-L1 therapies: Clinicopathological findings. *J Eur Acad Dermatol Venereol* 2017;31(10):e464–9.

103. Weber JS, Dummer R, de Pril V, Lebbe C, Hodi FS, MDX010-20 Investigators. Patterns of onset and resolution of immune-related adverse events of special interest with ipilimumab: Detailed safety analysis from a phase 3 trial in patients with advanced melanoma. *Cancer* 2013;119(9):1675–82.

104. Curry JL et al. Diverse types of dermatologic toxicities from immune checkpoint blockade therapy. *J Cutan Pathol* 2017;44(2):158–76.

105. Freeman-Keller M, Kim Y, Cronin H, Richards A, Gibney G, Weber JS. Nivolumab in resected and unresectable metastatic melanoma: Characteristics of immune-related adverse events and association with outcomes. *Clin Cancer Res* 2016;22(4):886–94.

106. Goldinger SM et al. Cytotoxic cutaneous adverse drug reactions during anti-PD-1 therapy. *Clin Cancer Res* 2016;22(16):4023–9.

107. Weber JS, Kahler KC, Hauschild A. Management of immune-related adverse events and kinetics of response with ipilimumab. *J Clin Oncol* 2012;30(21):2691–7.

108. Jour G et al. Autoimmune dermatologic toxicities from immune checkpoint blockade with anti-PD-1 antibody therapy: A report on bullous skin eruptions. *J Cutan Pathol* 2016;43(8):688–96.

109. Nayar N, Briscoe K, Fernandez Penas P. Toxic epidermal necrolysis-like reaction with severe satellite cell necrosis associated with nivolumab in a patient with ipilimumab refractory metastatic melanoma. *J Immunother* 2016;39(3):149–52.

110. Johnson DB et al. Severe cutaneous and neurologic toxicity in melanoma patients during vemurafenib administration following anti-PD-1 therapy. *Cancer Immunol Res* 2013;1(6):373–7.

111. Voskens CJ et al. The price of tumor control: An analysis of rare side effects of anti-CTLA-4 therapy in metastatic melanoma from the ipilimumab network. *PLoS One* 2013;8(1):e53745.

112. Wong RK et al. Clinical practice guidelines for the prevention and treatment of acute and late radiation reactions from the MASCC skin toxicity study group. *Support Care Cancer* 2013;21(10):2933–48.

113. Shaitelman SF et al. Acute and short-term toxic effects of conventionally fractionated vs hypofractionated whole-breast irradiation: A randomized clinical trial. *JAMA Oncol* 2015;1(7):931–41.

114. Hymes SR, Alousi AM, Cowen EW. Graft-versus-host disease: Part I. Pathogenesis and clinical manifestations of graft-versus-host disease. *J Am Acad Dermatol* 2012;66(4):515.e1–18, quiz 33–4.

115. Villarreal CD, Alanis JC, Perez JC, Candiani JO. Cutaneous graft-versus-host disease after hematopoietic stem cell transplant: A review. *Anais Brasileiros de Dermatologia* 2016;91(3):336–43.

2

Acneiform Eruptions

Gabriella Fabbrocini, Maria Concetta Romano, Sara Cacciapuoti, and Luigia Panariello

Background

Acneiform eruptions are defined as dermatoses that can be similar to acne vulgaris. Lesions may be papulopustular, nodular, or cystic. Acneiform eruptions usually lack comedones, whereas acne vulgaris typically consists of comedones. In this chapter we will focus on anti-EGFR inhibitor (EGFRi)–induced acneiform eruption, which is one of the most frequent dermatologic side effects occurring in oncologic patients, treated with these innovative drugs. The EGFRis most frequently responsible of acneiform eruption and their mechanism of action are listed in Table 2.1.

Considering their mechanism of action and the pleiotropic EGFR distribution in human skin, it is not surprising that both antibodies and tyrosine kinase inhibitors are able to cause acneiform eruptions with a high frequency (80%). This drug eruption is the most common cutaneous adverse event during EGFRi therapy; it has been reported to occur in 50–100% of patients (1–4).

Acneiform rash is a dose-dependent skin drug reaction, which usually develops in the first 1–2 weeks and peaks at 3–4 weeks on therapy. Inflamed papules and pustules, accompanied by itching in seborrheic regions, are characteristic findings. The development of this event after the EGFR inhibitor therapy was suggested to be a prognostic factor indicating good treatment response (5). This condition can affect the quality of life of these patients and it can sometimes lead to a discontinuation of the antineoplastic therapy.

Pathogenesis

EGFRis inhibit both EGFR in tumor cells and in normal cells of the epidermis. Inhibition of EGFR in keratinocytes induces apoptosis, arrests cell growth, reduces cell migration, and increases cell adhesivity and cell differentiation (Figure 2.1). The arrest of cell growth, migration of keratinocytes, and inflammation result in xerosis and acneiform rash.

Clinical Presentation

Patients with acneiform eruptions present with acnelike lesions such as papules and pustules. The skin reaction generally resolves without sequelae. Among the complications of acneiform rash, impetiginization is frequent. A bacterial impetiginization should be suspected when a sudden worsening of the rash (more polymorphous lesions and characteristic honey-colored crust) occurs. The major bacterium responsible for the impetiginization is *Staphylococcus aureus*, especially in patients with nasal carriage and truncal involvement (Figures 2.2 through 2.6) (6).

TABLE 2.1

EGFRis Most Frequently Responsible for Acneiform Eruption and Their Mechanism of Action

Drug's Molecular Structure	Drug's Denomination	Mechanism of Action
Monoclonal antibodies	Cetuximab (Erbitux®) Panitumumab (Vectibix®) Necitumumab	Binds the EGFR extracellularly, preventing its activation
Small molecule	Gefitinib (Iressa®) Erlotinib (Tarceva®) Afatinib (Gilotrif®) Dacomitinib Lapatinib (Tykerb®) Osimertinib (Tagrisso®)	Inhibits the intracellular tyrosine kinase domain of EGFR, preventing activation of downstream signaling cascades

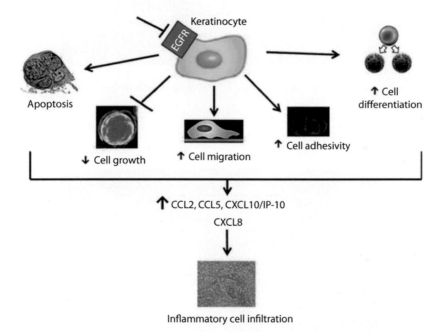

FIGURE 2.1   Pathogenesis of inflammatory cell infiltration occurring in the EGFRi-induced papulopustular rash.

Histology

In biopsy specimens taken from affected areas, the stratum corneum is noted to be thinner and more compact, with occasional focal parakeratosis and loss of normal basket-weave configuration, together with slight hypogranulosis, prominent keratin plugs, and dilated follicular infundibula (7).

Therapy

Different therapeutic strategies and recommendations have been proposed based on case reports, clinical experience, consensus, or randomized studies with small sample sizes (1,8). This could be a consequence of the difficulty in recruiting a large number of patients with such specific characteristics for trials.

Treatment should be personalized depending on the severity of the rash (Table 2.2) (9–11). As prophylactic therapy, oral antibiotics with anti-inflammatory effects (doxycycline 100–200 mg/day), or antihistamines can be used along with topical steroids. Many products should be avoided for their irritating

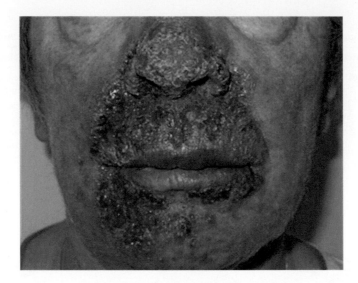

FIGURE 2.2   Acneiform rash of the face in a patient treated with panitumumab for colorectal cancer, grade 2.

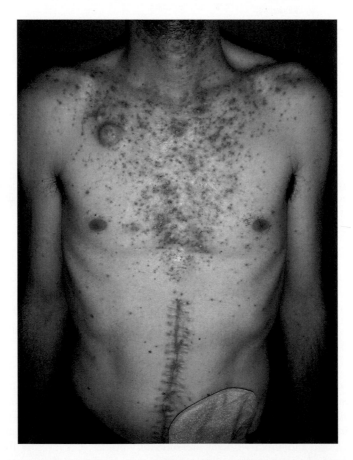

FIGURE 2.3   Acneiform rash of the trunk in a patient treated with panitumumab + fluorouracil and irinotecan, grade 2.

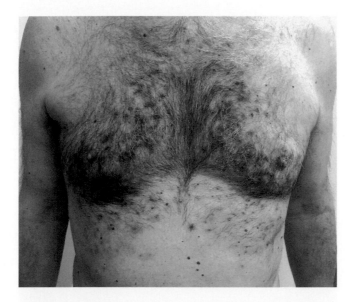

FIGURE 2.4 Secondary infection in a patient treated with afatinib.

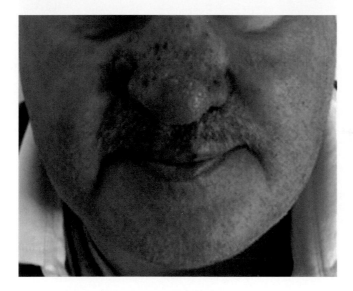

FIGURE 2.5 Acneiform rash in a patient treated with erlotinib, grade 1.

effects: benzoyl peroxide and retinoids. Patients should avoid direct sunlight exposure or sunbathing, and hot or humid environments. Greasy creams such as petroleum jelly have high effective properties, but, on the other hand, their occlusive characteristics may lead to folliculitis.

When the rash reaches grade 2, it is recommended to use topical corticosteroids (hydrocortisone 2.5% cream) (12). However, in our experience and as already reported in other studies, patients may benefit from topical clindamycin or erythromycin. If the patient complains of itching, topical menthol cream or an oral antihistamine can be used. We can add oral tetracycline for the anti-inflammatory effect (minocycline 100 mg/day, lymecycline 300 mg/day, or doxycycline 100 mg/day) (12,13). Low-dose isotretinoin is also suggested (12).

When the acneiform rash is severe (grade 3 or 4), high doses of oral tetracyclines (minocycline 2 × 100 mg/day, lymecycline 2 × 300 mg/day, or doxycycline 2 × 100 mg/day) should be added to the

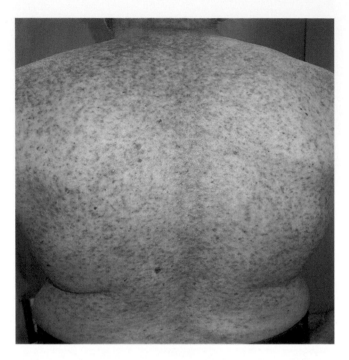

FIGURE 2.6   Acneiform rash in a patient treated with gefitinib, grade 2.

previous therapies. When the acute phase vanishes, the treatment can be tapered. In case of suspected superinfection, bacteriological and/or viral tests (e.g., swabs) should be performed and, if necessary, appropriate oral or intravenous antibiotics. Oral corticosteroids (oral prednisone 0.5 mg/kg for 5 days) can be considered, too (12).

In grade 3 and 4 rashes, when toxicities are not reduced after 2–4 weeks, despite treatment, dose reduction or discontinuation of EGFRis should be taken into consideration as it may be required.

TABLE 2.2

Therapy of EGFRi-Induced Folliculitis, According to Grade

	Prevention	**Grade 1**	**Grade 2**	**Grades 3–4**
Pharmacological treatment	Oral antibiotics (doxycycline 100–200 mg/day) and antihistamines	Oral tetracycline (minocycline 100 mg/day, lymecycline 300 mg/day or doxycycline 100 mg/day), additional to supporting precautions	Topical corticosteroids, such as hydrocortisone 2.5% cream	High doses of oral tetracyclines (minocycline 2 × 100 mg/day, lymecycline 2 × 300 mg/day, or doxycycline 2 × 100 mg/day) Oral corticosteroids (oral prednisone 0.5 mg/kg for 5 days), additional to the therapy described for grade 2 If toxicities are not reduced after 2–4 weeks, despite treatment, dose reduction or discontinuation of EGFRi may be necessary If superinfection suspected: bacteriological and/or viral swab
Supporting skin care products	Emollient and moisturizing cream Perfume-free cleanser with a pH of 5.5 Photoprotection Therapeutic makeup	Same skin care products	Same skin care products	Same skin care products

Besides the pharmacological treatment, it is necessary to recommend a specific dermocosmetological protocol for all patients treated with EGFRis, as the modified cellular turnover and the damaged corneal barrier can take advantage of cosmetical management. In our experience, the dermocosmetological protocol should be prescribed at the beginning of cancer therapy. This protocol aims to make the skin "unsusceptible" to EGFR inhibition–induced processes by the action of substances mimicking EGFR functions (vegetable fats or chemical fats combined with antioxidant molecules).

Moreover, it is fundamental to restore the integrity and the water balance of the epidermal barrier to treat the xerosis associated with acneiform rashes thanks to the following precautions: using formulations without water (oil, ointment, and cream) and choosing vegetable fats over mineral fats, as these support the biochemical affinity between skin and dermocosmetological substances. Patients' skin routines should concern cleansing, hydration, and restoration, preferring alcohol-free, ointment–oil formulations.

A broad-spectrum sunscreen should be prescribed during spring and summer seasons.

To reduce the impact on quality of life of skin manifestation of grades 1 and 2 rashes, a specific nonocclusive makeup could be used, which is usually well tolerated by all patients. In order to protect the stratum corneum barrier, cosmetic formulations containing fatty acids and ceramides are recommended.

Dermatologists should be aware of signs of superinfection, especially bacterial ones from *Staphylococcus aureus*, but also fungal and viral infections could be possible. In case of doubt, a skin swab should be performed.

It is interesting that >30% of all the patients treated with EGFRis, who developed a cutaneous bacterial, viral, or fungal superinfection of the papulopustular rash, were colonized with *S. aureus* in the nasopharyngeal cavity, as opposed to only 2.2% in whom no dermatological infection was documented. For this reason the use of intranasal mupirocin has been recommended in patients with papulopustular rash to prevent the risk of secondary infection.

Prevention

Preventive therapy is essential in patients treated with EGFRis and can prevent and reduce the severity of skin reactions. Taking care of patients at the beginning of the oncotherapy, before adverse events appear, is the right choice to avoid rash or otherwise to manage it.

Patients should be informed of the specific cutaneous adverse events before starting the therapy. Patients should also be advised to minimize their exposure to sunlight because rash may be more severe in sun-exposed areas of the skin. They should also avoid soap with a basic pH and alcohol-based fragrances and lotions. Patients' skin routines should be the same of that described in the "Therapy" section.

Several studies show that oral antibiotics can be prescribed as prophylactic therapy, in particular the tetracycline class such as doxycycline (100–200 mg/day) or minocycline (100 mg/day) (12).

This class of antibiotics, in fact, has anti-inflammatory and tissue-protective effects. Doxycycline is a safe option in patients with renal dysfunction, while minocycline is appropriate during summer or in regions with a high UV index, because it is less photosensitizing (14).

Antibiotic administration should begin at the first day of starting EGFRi treatment, because toxicity can arise as early as 2 days after the first dose. Nevertheless, in our experience preventive therapy can reduce the incidence and the grade of acneiform rash and allows dermatologists to avoid the use of systemic antibiotics, which should be necessary only in case of resistance to topical therapy or in case of superinfection.

Differential Diagnosis

Bacterial Folliculitis

The EGFRi papulopustular rash can be complicated by bacterial superinfection, especially from *S. aureus*. Folliculitis can appear similar to papulopustular eruption, thus it can be misdiagnosed.

Rarely a delay in starting antibiotic therapy can lead to bloodstream infection, in particular in immune-compromised patients.

Physicians can use two characteristics to distinguish between papulopustular rash and bacterial folliculitis: location and timing (15). The following locations are suspected for superinfection: upper and lower extremities, lower abdomen, buttocks, and groin. The appearance of a new rash after 12 weeks of EGFRi therapy, regardless of location, is suspicious for a bacterial superinfection.

Conclusions

Acneiform rash is the most common cutaneous adverse event caused by EGFRis. As the use of EGFRis increases, it will be fundamental to diagnose and manage this adverse effect, especially to ensure patient's compliance and adherence to oncological therapy.

Studies are needed to better understand the pathogenetic mechanism and the histologic modification occurring in papulopustular rash in order to develop new standardized therapeutic and preventive measures.

REFERENCES

1. Chanprapaph K, Vachiramon V, Rattanakaemakorn P. Epidermal growth factor receptor inhibitors: A review of cutaneous adverse events and management. *Dermatol Res Pract* 2014;2014:734249.
2. Segaert S, Van Custem E. Clinical signs, pathophysiology and management of skin toxicity during therapy with epidermal growth factor receptor inhibitors. *Ann Oncol* 2005;16(9):1425–33.
3. Jacot W et al. Acneiform eruption induced by epidermal growth factor receptor inhibitors in patients with solid tumours. *Br J Dermatol* 2004;151:238–41.
4. Ha KD, Navid E, Wolverton ES. Drug induced acneiform eruptions. In: Zeichner JA, ed. *Acneiform Eruptions in Dermatology.* 1st ed. New York, NY: Springer-Verlag; 2014; pp. 389–404.
5. Journagan S, Obadiah J. An acneiform eruption due to erlotinib: Prognostic implications and management. *J Am Acad Dermatol* 2006;54:358–60.
6. Peuvrel L, Bachmeyer C, Reguiai Z, Bachet JB, André T, Bensadoun RJ et al. Semiology of skin toxicity associated with epidermal growth factor receptor (EGFR) inhibitors. *Support Care Cancer* 2012;20:909–21.
7. Vanhoefer U, Tewes M, Rojo F, Dirsch O, Schleucher N, Rosen O et al. Phase I study of the humanized antiepidermal growth factor receptor monoclonal antibody EMD72000 in patients with advanced solid tumors that express the epidermal growth factor receptor. *J Clin Oncol* 2004;22:175–84.
8. Liu S, Kurzrock R. Understanding toxicities of targeted agents: Implications for anti-tumor activity and management. *Semin Oncol* 2015 Dec;42(6):863–75.
9. Dreno B, Bensadoun RJ, Humbert P, Krutmann J, Luger T, Triller R et al. Algorithm for dermocosmetic use in the management of cutaneous side-effects associated with targeted therapy in oncology. *J Eur Acad Dermatol Venereol* 2013;27:1071–80.
10. Liu S, Kurzrock R. Understanding toxicities of targeted agents: Implications for anti-tumor activity and management. *Semin Oncol* 2015;42:863–75.
11. Hofheinz RD, Deplanque G, Komatsu Y, Kobayashi Y, Ocvirk J, Racca P et al. Recommendations for the prophylactic management of skin reactions induced by epidermal growth factor receptor inhibitors in patients with solid tumors. *Oncologist* 2016;21:1483–491.
12. Lacouture ME, Anadkat M, Jatoi A, Garawin T, Bohac C, Mitchell E. Dermatologic toxicity occurring during anti-EGFR monoclonal inhibitor therapy in patients with metastatic colorectal cancer: A systematic review. *Clin Colorectal Cancer* 2018;17(2):85–96.
13. Grande R, Narducci F, Bianchetti S, Mansueto G, Gemma D, Sperduti I et al. Pre-emptive skin toxicity treatment for anti-EGFR drugs: Evaluation of efficacy of skin moisturizers and lymecycline. A phase II study. *Support Care Cancer* 2013;21(6):1691–695.
14. Stulhofer Buzina D, Martinac I, Ledic DD, Ceovic R, Bilic I, Marinovic B. The most common cutaneous side effects of epidermal growth factor receptor inhibitors and their management. *Acta Dermatovenerol Croat* 2015;23:282–88.
15. Braden R, Anadkat M. EGFR inhibitor-induced skin reactions: Differentiating acneiform rash from superimposed bacterial infections. *Support Care Cancer* 2016;24:3943–950.

3

Hair Disorders

Azael Freites-Martinez, Gabriella Fabbrocini, Mario E. Lacouture, and Antonella Tosti

Introduction

The most commonly encountered hair disorder in cancer patients is chemotherapy-induced alopecia (CIA) (1). However, several other anticancer therapies can also be associated with alopecia and other hair disorders, including radiotherapy, targeted therapy, immunotherapy, stem cell transplants, and hormonal therapies. In addition, alteration in hair growth, pigmentation, and texture may also be encountered, although they have not been systematically documented in cancer patients. Childhood and breast cancer survivors are at an increased risk for persistent or permanent alopecia with frequencies as high as 14% (2) and 30% (3), respectively. Survivors with persistent or permanent alopecia are more likely to identify role limitations owing to emotional problems, which may suggest an impact from negative self-esteem or self-image (2).

This chapter reviews the types of hair disorders attributed to anticancer therapies in cancer patients and survivors, and offers adequate management of these conditions.

Hair Disorders Induced by Traditional Anticancer Therapies

Cytotoxic Chemotherapy

Chemotherapy-Induced Alopecia

CIA usually begins within days to weeks after the first dose of cytotoxic chemotherapy as a nonscarring, patchy, or diffuse anagen effluvium with predominance in areas of increased friction, such as crown and temporo-occipital areas, that may progress to complete alopecia in 2–3 months. A Korean study suggests that anagen effluvium induced by chemotherapy does not affect the scalp uniformly, but rather it is less severe along occipital hairlines in men and frontal hairlines in females (4). In addition to scalp alopecia, alopecia of other body areas could be observed. Trichoscopic findings in CIA are those of anagen effluvium, including black dots, yellow dots, exclamation mark hairs, and color and thickness hair shaft changes (Figure 3.1). Although the clinical manifestation of CIA from different drugs seems similar (Table 3.1), accumulating evidence suggests that the molecular underpinnings are varied and are subject to the individual's susceptibility (5).

Persistent Chemotherapy-Induced Alopecia

Persistent chemotherapy-induced alopecia (pCIA), also known as permanent alopecia after chemotherapy, is the persistence of CIA after 6 months of chemotherapy discontinuation, observed in up to 30% of breast cancer survivors (3) and up to 14% in childhood cancer survivors (2). pCIA has been mostly observed in breast cancer survivors treated with taxane-based chemotherapy regimens (paclitaxel and docetaxel) (6), in combination with other chemotherapies (such as cyclophosphamide, thiotepa, and carboplatin), in pediatric patients who have undergone a conditioning regimen with busulfan (alone or in combination with cyclophosphamide) for bone marrow transplantation (7) (Table 3.1), and radiation.

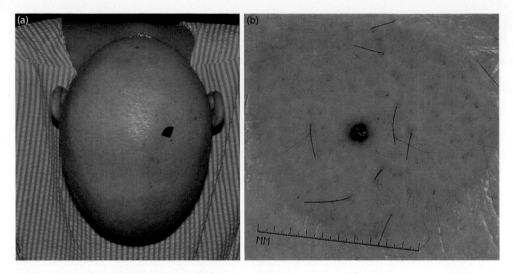

FIGURE 3.1   Chemotherapy-induced alopecia. (a) Clinical aspect after 6 weeks of the first dose of docetaxel. (b) Trichoscopy: black and yellow dots and broken hairs.

TABLE 3.1

Anticancer Therapies Commonly Causing Reversible or Persistent Alopecia

Anticancer Therapy	Tumor Types Indicated or under Investigation	Incidence (%) of Reversible Alopecia	Incidence (%) of Persistent Alopecia
Chemotherapies			
Cyclophosphamide	Breast cancer, leukemia, lymphoma, multiple myeloma, neuroblastoma, retinoblastoma, ovarian cancer	25 (low dose), ~100 (high dose)	Reported predominantly with taxane-based chemotherapy (30%)
Daunorubicin, doxorubicin, and idarubicin	AML, ALL, thyroid cancer, breast cancer, gastric cancer, lung cancer, bladder cancer, lymphomas, neuroblastoma, sarcomas, Wilms tumor	~100	
Taxanes (docetaxel, paclitaxel)	Breast cancer, gastric cancer, head and neck cancer, lung cancer, prostate cancer	~100	30
Etoposide	Small cell lung cancer, testicular cancer	~55	
Irinotecan and topotecan	Colorectal cancer, small cell lung cancer, ovarian cancer, cervical cancer	~50	
Radiotherapy			
Photon radiotherapy (traditional radiotherapy) and proton radiotherapy	Primary CNS tumors, brain metastasis, head and neck cancer	75–100	Up to 50% risk with high-fractionated follicular dose of 43 Gy (photon radiotherapy)

(*Continued*)

TABLE 3.1 (*Continued*)

Anticancer Therapies Commonly Causing Reversible or Persistent Alopecia

Anticancer Therapy	Tumor Types Indicated or under Investigation	Incidence (%) of Reversible Alopecia	Incidence (%) of Persistent Alopecia
Targeted Therapies			
Vismodegib	Basal cell carcinoma (locally advanced or unresectable)	62	Rarely reported
Sorafenib	Hepatocellular carcinoma, renal cell carcinoma, thyroid cancer	26	
Sunitinib and regorafenib	Metastatic renal cell carcinoma, gastrointestinal stromal tumor	4–6	
Vemurafenib and dabrafenib	Melanoma (stage IV)	19–24	
Immunotherapies			
CTLA-4	Melanoma (stages III–IV)	1–2	
PD-1 and PD-L1	Melanoma (stage IV), lung, Hodgkin lymphoma, urothelial carcinoma	2	
Stem Cell Transplants			
Conditioning chemotherapy (busulfan, topotecan, thiotepa, etoposide, cyclophosphamide)	Leukemia	~100	30
Graft-versus-host disease		20	20
Endocrine Therapies			
Leuprolide	Breast cancer,	2	~25 in breast cancer survivors
Octreotide	hepatocellular carcinoma, neuroendocrine tumors	6.7	
Aromatase inhibitors (anastrozole, letrozole, exemestane)	Metastatic estrogen receptor–positive (ER+) breast cancer	~25	

Abbreviations: AML, acute myelogenous leukemia; ALL, acute lymphocytic leukemia; CTLA-4, cytotoxic T-lymphocyte-associated protein 4; PD-1, programmed cell death protein 1; PD-L1, programmed death-ligand 1; ~, approximately.

Multiple clinical features have been described for pCIA (Table 3.2). The most common is diffuse nonscarring alopecia with hair changes involving the hair strength, texture, length, and color (Figure 3.2). The alopecia is often more severe on androgen-dependent scalp and can be misdiagnosed as androgenetic alopecia (Figure 3.3). pCIA can also affect the axilla, pubic area, eyelashes, and eyebrows. As seen in other alopecias, clinical features are nonspecific and a complete medical history, including a total body examination, is needed to determine the offending therapy or any other possible alopecia etiology. Dystrophic and miniaturized hairs may be seen in trichoscopy (Figure 3.4).

Histopathologic features of permanent or persistent alopecia attributed to anticancer therapies are characterized by a severe reduction in the total number of hair follicles in the absence of fibrosis. Other features of pCIA include an increased number of miniaturized and telogen hair follicles (8), as well as increased numbers of fibrous streamers (stelae) in both the reticular dermis and subcutis (9,10). Other, less

TABLE 3.2

Clinical Features of Hair Disorders Attributed to Anticancer Therapies

Anticancer Therapy	Clinical Features

Chemotherapies	Alopecia—Nonscarring, predominantly anagen effluvium on areas of increased friction at the beginning. Usually totally recovered after 6 months of last chemotherapy cycle. Alopecia of other body areas are usually observed. Trichoscopy is not specific: black dots, yellow dots, exclamation mark hairs, and color and thickness changes along the hair may exist.
	Pigmentary and textural hair changes—Hypo- and hyperpigmentation. Straight hair may become curly or wavy, and finer, usually resolving 6 months after last chemotherapy cycle.
	Hirsutism—May be observed, predominantly on the face.
	Persistent chemotherapy-induced alopecia:
	   Diffuse hair thinning is reported. A similar pattern to androgenetic alopecia is also described. Changes are mostly based on hair thinning.
	   Scarring features have been reported.
	   Other body areas may be involved.

Radiotherapies	Alopecia—Nonscarring alopecia is described; geometric shapes in relation with the irradiated area. Radiation dermatitis might be present. Trichoscopy is not specific, including yellow and black dots, short vellus hair, peripilar sign and broken hair. Pigmentary and textural hair changes—Hair hypopigmentation and decreased shaft diameter may be seen. Persistent radiotherapy-induced alopecia—Features of scarring alopecia are frequent, with atrophic skin and scarce hairs in severe cases. Diffuse hair thinning in total cranial irradiation and in combination with cytotoxic chemotherapy.
Targeted therapies	Alopecia—Diffuse alopecia with nonscarring and scarring features after severe inflammatory follicular reactions (e.g., erosive pustular dermatosis of the scalp, tufted hair folliculitis). Hirsutism, hypertrichosis, and trichomegaly—Hirsutism and periocular hypertrichosis especially in women. Eyelash and eyebrow hypertrichosis is frequent, with long and curly eyelashes that may affect vision (predominantly with EGFR inhibitors). Pigmentary and textural hair changes—Hair discoloration, including hypopigmentation (VEGFR/PDGFR) and hyperpigmentation (EGFR inhibitors).
Immunotherapies	Alopecia—Diffuse hair thinning and alopecia areata. Pigmentary hair changes—Hyper- and hypopigmentation can be seen.
Stem cell transplants	Alopecia—Scarring alopecia similar as described for chemotherapies, related to conditioning chemotherapies; alopecia areata with graft-versus-host disease. Pigmentary and textural hair changes—Hypopigmentation and hair thinning. Persistent hair changes—Diffuse alopecia with scarring features could be observed (similar to persistent chemotherapy-induced alopecia).
Vismodegib	Alopecia—Similar as described for chemotherapies. Persistent hair changes—Persistent alopecia has been rarely reported (similar to persistent chemotherapy-induced alopecia).
Endocrine therapies	Alopecia—Pattern alopecia, similar to androgenetic type. Hirsutism—Hirsutism may be observed.

Abbreviations: EGFR, epidermal growth factor receptor inhibitor; VEGFR, vascular endothelial growth factor receptor; PDGFR, platelet-derived growth factor receptor.

typically reported histopathologic features of pCIA include a pattern of scarring alopecia, with concentric fibrosis and a discrete lymphoid cell infiltrate around the follicles (10) (Figure 3.4).

Radiotherapy

Radiotherapy-Induced Alopecia

Radiotherapy-induced alopecia (RIA) is characterized by an anagen effluvium followed by telogen shedding for a premature catagen entry of follicles. A geometrical-shape alopecia patch confined to the area of radiotherapy is usually observed 1–3 weeks after the first irradiation (Table 3.2) and complete

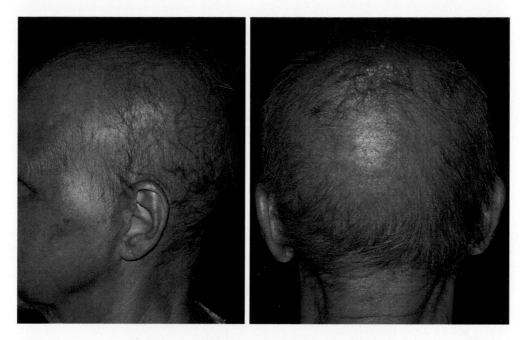

FIGURE 3.2 Persistent chemotherapy-induced alopecia: diffuse hair thinning and hair discoloration. Clinical aspect after 3 years of the last cycle of taxane chemotherapy.

hair regrowth usually occurs 2–4 months after radiotherapy. Other dermatologic adverse events may be observed in up to 45% of cases, including erythema, radiation dermatitis, and ulcers, which may need additional attention in the acute phase (11) (Figure 3.5). Yellow and black dots have been described as the predominant trichoscopic findings in 60% of RIA, followed by short vellus hair, peripilar sign, and broken hair (12).

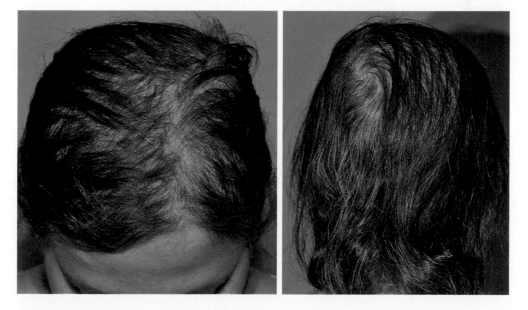

FIGURE 3.3 Persistent chemotherapy-induced alopecia: similar pattern to androgenetic alopecia. Clinical aspect after 18 months of the last cycle of taxane chemotherapy.

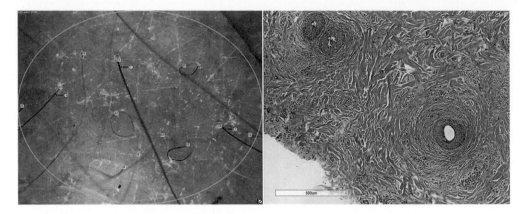

FIGURE 3.4 Persistent chemotherapy-induced alopecia. Trichoscopy: predominance of one hair per follicular unit with vellus and dystrophic hairs. Histopathology (H&E, 500 microns): reduction in total number of hair follicles with mild perifollicular lymphocytic inflammation and fibrosis.

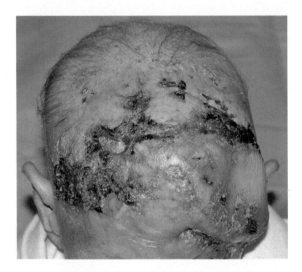

FIGURE 3.5 Radiotherapy-induced alopecia. Scalp alopecia with ulcers and crusts after photon radiotherapy (traditional radiotherapy).

Persistent Radiotherapy-Induced Alopecia

Persistent radiotherapy-induced alopecia (pRIA) is defined as the incomplete hair regrowth 6 months following therapy cessation. This is commonly related to high-dose radiotherapy to the scalp (usually >30 Gy with photon radiotherapy, and >21 Gy with proton radiotherapy). Clinical presentation of pRIA includes well-defined, usually asymptomatic alopecic and atrophic skin confined to the area of radiotherapy (Figure 3.6). Telogen hair follicles are not usually affected if the radiation dose is low, therefore alopecia may be not complete (13).

Endocrine Therapies

Endocrine Therapy–Induced Alopecia and Hirsutism

A meta-analysis of endocrine therapy–induced alopecia (EIA) reported an overall incidence of all-grade alopecia of 4.4% and high-grade alopecia (more than 50% of hair loss) of 1.2%, with the highest incidence of all-grade alopecia (25.4%) observed in patients treated with tamoxifen (14).

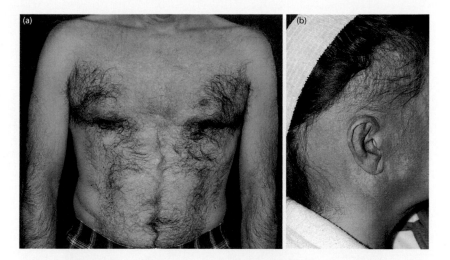

FIGURE 3.6 Persistent radiotherapy-induced alopecia and hair changes. (a) Trunk alopecia and hair graying after mantle radiation. (b) Persistent alopecia after scalp radiation on the temporal area.

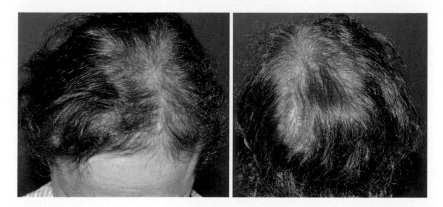

FIGURE 3.7 Endocrine therapy–induced alopecia: similar pattern to androgenetic alopecia. Clinical aspect after 12 months of therapy with anastrozole.

The mean time to alopecia development is 17 months (15,16). These patients usually present with recession of frontal and parietal hairlines (Table 3.2), mimicking the typical pattern of androgenetic alopecia (Figure 3.7). Trichoscopic features observed in patients with EIA include the features of androgenetic alopecia (Figure 3.8). Iatrogenic hirsutism has been reported in patients receiving endocrine therapy (ET) for breast cancer (17).

In patients treated with cytotoxic chemotherapy followed by ET, a complete medical history must be obtained to define whether alopecia is attributed to the actual ET (EIA) or to the previous chemotherapy (pCIA), or even the combination of both therapies (pCIA + EIA).

Targeted Therapies, Immunotherapies, and Stem Cell Transplant

Alopecia, and Textural and Pigmentary Hair Changes

Alopecia

Whereas mild alopecia is frequent with epidermal growth factor receptor (EGFR) inhibitors (e.g., erlotinib, afatinib, cetuximab, panitumumab), scarring alopecia has been reported in 5% of patients treated with

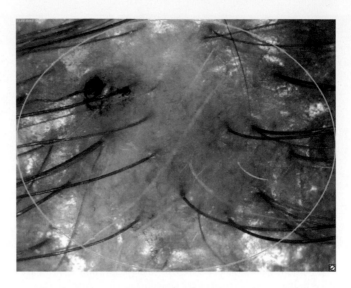

FIGURE 3.8 Endocrine therapy–induced alopecia: trichoscopy features of the crown area showing the predominance of one hair per follicular unit and multiple vellus hairs.

cetuximab, which may be a consequence of a secondary folliculitis (Figure 3.9). Alopecia areata and universalis are considered immune-related adverse effects (AEs) occurring in around 5% of patients receiving the cytotoxic T-lymphocyte antigen 4 (CTLA-4) inhibitor ipilimumab (18). With the (PD-1 inhibitor) nivolumab, there is a reported incidence of 1% of alopecia not otherwise specified. Vismodegib (19) has been reported to cause alopecia in 62% of patients; persistent alopecia after vismodegib cessation may be observed, which is clinically characterized by a diffuse pattern.

Among patients undergoing stem cell transplantation, diffuse alopecia is reported in association with conditioning chemotherapy in around 100% of recipients and with similar features as described in CIA. Hair changes may occur with graft-versus-host disease: in the acute setting, features include nonscarring alopecia with diffuse hair thinning, patchy hair loss, and premature graying. Alopecia areata and other autoimmune skin conditions such as vitiligo have been reported. Chronic graft-versus-host disease after stem cell transplant may induce both diffuse alopecia and permanent alopecia with features resembling lichen planopilaris (20) (Table 3.2).

Textural and Pigmentary Hair Changes

Textural and pigmentary hair changes are usually temporary, until the follicular unit begins regularly functioning again (Figure 3.10). Pigmentary hair changes include depigmentation (Figure 3.11) and repigmentation, most apparent on the scalp. Hair hypopigmentation has been reported with the multikinase inhibitors (pazopanib, sunitinib, regorafenib), whereas EGFR inhibitors result in hyperpigmentation of scalp and facial hair (~50%). Additionally, hair repigmentation has been described as a possible marker of good tumor response in patients receiving anti-PD-1/anti–PD-L1 therapy for lung cancer (21). Excessive hair growth over the periocular area, hirsutism, and trichomegaly (Figure 3.12) have been mostly reported as an AE with EGFR inhibitors (22–24).

Clinical Grading of Hair Disorders in Cancer Patients

Numerous instruments in the oncology literature exist to objectify the grade of the hair disorder. Of all these grading instruments, the Common Terminology Criteria for Adverse Events (CTCAE v5.0) is the most utilized standard for the description of drug safety in cancer treatments (Table 3.3). However, other grading instruments include the World Health Organization (WHO), Dean scale, the National

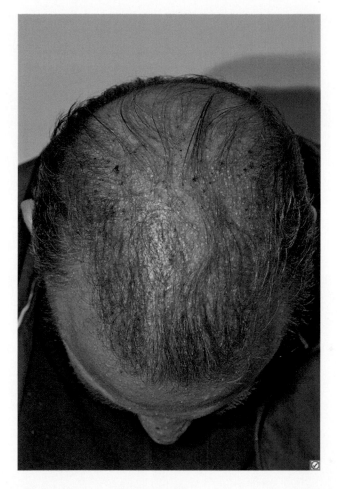

FIGURE 3.9   Scalp folliculitis in a patient receiving cetuximab.

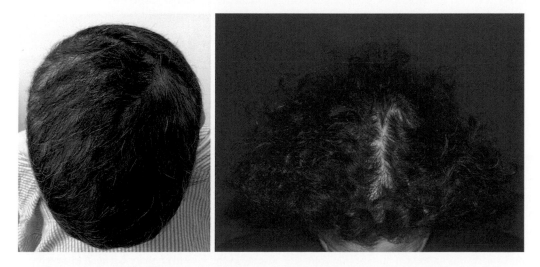

FIGURE 3.10   Transitory hair texture changes after doxorubicin and cyclophosphamide chemotherapy.

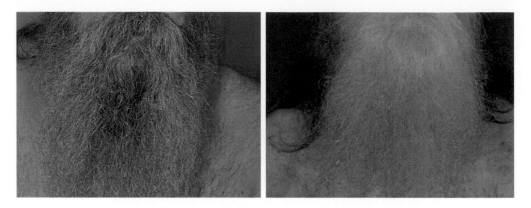

FIGURE 3.11   Hair depigmentation in a patient receiving ipilimumab/nivolumab.

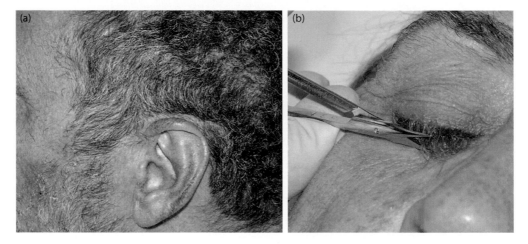

FIGURE 3.12   (a) Hypertrichosis in a patient receiving erlotinib. (b) Eyelash hypertrichosis in a patient receiving erlotinib. Eyelash and eyebrow clipping, and referral to an ophthalmologist are indicated for patients with ocular symptoms.

Cancer Institute (NCI), and the EGFR Inhibitor Skin Toxicity Tool (Table 3.3). For eyelash and eyebrow alopecia, there are no validated grading scales; however, hypertrichosis and trichomegaly are graded with the CTCAE v5.0 (25). The modified Ferriman-Gallwey scoring system may also be used to grade hypertrichosis (26).

Conclusion

Anticancer therapy–induced hair disorders have a significant impact on cancer patients' quality of life. Accumulating evidence suggests that the molecular underpinnings of alopecia are varied and are subject to individual susceptibility, yet they do appear to activate or share several molecular damage-response pathways. Prevention of chemotherapy-induced alopecia using scalp cooling appears to offer the most promising results to prevent this specific untoward adverse event. However, there is a need to develop hair follicle stem cell–reactive management and individualized risk-prediction strategies.

TABLE 3.3

Grading Scales Used for Anticancer Therapy–Induced Hair Changes

Grade 1	Grade 2	Grade 3	Grade 4
Alopecia Grading			
CTCAE v5.0			
Hair loss of <50% of normal for that individual that is not obvious from a distance but only on close inspection; a different hairstyle may be required to cover the hair loss, but it does not require a wig or hairpiece to camouflage.	Hair loss of ≥50% normal for that individual that is readily apparent to others; a wig or hair piece is necessary if the patient desires to completely camouflage the hair loss; associated with psychosocial impact.	–	–
Dean Grading Scale of Hair Loss Protection from Anticancer Therapies			
>0–25% hair loss	25–50% hair loss	50–75% hair loss	75–100% hair loss
WHO Handbook for Reporting Results of Cancer Treatment			
Minimal hair loss	Moderate, patchy hair loss	Complete alopecia, but reversible	Nonreversible alopecia
EGFR Inhibitor Skin Toxicity Tool (MESTT)			
Hair loss <50% of normal for that individual that may or may not be noticeable to others but is associated with increased shedding and overall feeling of less volume. May require different hairstyle to cover but does not require hairpiece to camouflage.	2A: Hair loss associated with marked increase shedding and 50–74% loss compared to normal for that individual. Hair loss is apparent to others, may be difficult to camouflage with change in hairstyle, and may require a hairpiece. 2B: Marked loss of at least 75% hair compared to normal for that individual with inability to camouflage except with a full wig or new cicatricial hair loss documented by biopsy that covers at least 5% scalp surface area. May impact on functioning in social, personal, or professional situations.	–	–
Hypertrichosis Grading			
CTCAE v5.0			
Increase in length, thickness, or density of hair that the patient is either able to camouflage by periodic shaving or removal of hairs, or is not concerned enough about the overgrowth to use any form of hair removal.	Increase in length, thickness, or density of hair at least on the usual exposed areas of the body (face, not limited to beard/moustache area; plus/minus arms) that require frequent shaving or use of destructive means of hair removal to camouflage; associated with psychosocial impact.	–	–
Hirsutism Grading			
CTCAE v5.0			
In women, increase in length, thickness, or density of hair in a male distribution that the patient is able to camouflage by periodic shaving, bleaching, or removal of hair.	In women, increase in length, thickness, or density of hair in a male distribution that requires daily shaving or consistent destructive means of hair removal to camouflage; associated with psychosocial impact.	–	–

REFERENCES

1. Lemieux J, Maunsell E, Provencher L. Chemotherapy-induced alopecia and effects on quality of life among women with breast cancer: A literature review. *Psychooncology* 2008;17:317–28.
2. Kinahan KE et al. Scarring, disfigurement, and quality of life in long-term survivors of childhood cancer: A report from the Childhood Cancer Survivor study. *J Clin Oncol* 2012;30:2466–74.
3. Kang D et al. 80P—Incidence of permanent chemotherapy-induced alopecia among breast cancer patients: A five-year prospective cohort study. *Ann Oncol* 2017;28(Suppl 10).
4. Yun SJ, Kim SJ. Hair loss pattern due to chemotherapy-induced anagen effluvium: A cross-sectional observation. *Dermatology* 2007;215:36–40.
5. Paus R, Haslam IS, Sharov AA, Botchkarev VA. Pathobiology of chemotherapy-induced hair loss. *Lancet Oncol* 2013;14:e50–9.
6. Bourgeois HP et al. Long term persistent alopecia and suboptimal hair regrowth after adjuvant chemotherapy for breast cancer: Alert for an emerging side effect: French ALOPERS observatory. *Ann Oncol* 2010;21:viii83–4.
7. Sedlacek SM. Persistent significant alopecia (PSA) from adjuvant docetaxel after doxorubicin/cyclophosphamide (AC) chemotherapy in women with breast cancer. *Breast Cancer Res Treat* 2006;171(3):627–34, abstract no. 2105.
8. Basilio FM, Brenner FM, Werner B, Rastelli GJ. Clinical and histological study of permanent alopecia after bone marrow transplantation. *Anais Brasileiros de Dermatologia* 2015;90:814–21.
9. Miteva M, Misciali C, Fanti PA, Vincenzi C, Romanelli P, Tosti A. Permanent alopecia after systemic chemotherapy: A clinicopathological study of 10 cases. *Am J Dermatopathol* 2011;33:345–50.
10. Tosti A, Piraccini BM, Vincenzi C, Misciali C. Permanent alopecia after busulfan chemotherapy. *Br J Dermatol* 2005;152:1056–8.
11. Haruna F, Lipsett A, Marignol L. Topical management of acute radiation dermatitis in breast cancer patients: A systematic review and meta-analysis. *Anticancer Res* 2017;37:5343–53.
12. Mubki T, Rudnicka L, Olszewska M, Shapiro J. Evaluation and diagnosis of the hair loss patient: Part I. History and clinical examination. *J Am Acad Dermatol* 2014;71:415.e1–415.e15.
13. Freites-Martinez A et al. CME Part 2: Hair disorders in cancer survivors Persistent chemotherapy-induced alopecia, persistent radiotherapy-induced alopecia, and hair growth disorders related to endocrine therapy or cancer surgery. *J Am Acad Dermatol* 2018.
14. Saggar V, Wu S, Dickler MN, Lacouture ME. Alopecia with endocrine therapies in patients with cancer. *Oncologist* 2013;18:1126–34.
15. Freites-Martinez A et al. Endocrine therapy-induced alopecia in patients with breast cancer. *JAMA Dermatology* 2018;154(6):670–5.
16. Freites-Martinez A et al. Dermatologic adverse events in breast cancer patients receiving endocrine therapies. *J Clin Oncol* 2017;35(15):e12533.
17. Al-Niaimi F, Lyon C. Tamoxifen-induced hirsutism. *J Drugs Dermatol* 2011;10:799–801.
18. Yamazaki N et al. Phase II study of ipilimumab monotherapy in Japanese patients with advanced melanoma. *Cancer Chemother Pharmacol* 2015;76:997–1004.
19. Alkeraye S, Maire C, Desmedt E, Templier C, Mortier L. Persistent alopecia induced by vismodegib. *Br J Dermatol* 2015;172:1671–2.
20. Harries MJ et al. How not to get scar(r)ed: Pointers to the correct diagnosis in patients with suspected primary cicatricial alopecia. *Br J Dermatol* 2009;160:482–501.
21. Rivera N et al. Hair repigmentation during immunotherapy treatment with an anti-programmed cell death 1 and anti-programmed cell death ligand 1 agent for lung cancer. *JAMA Dermatology* 2017;153(11):1162–5.
22. Dueland S, Sauer T, Lund-Johansen F, Ostenstad B, Tveit KM. Epidermal growth factor receptor inhibition induces trichomegaly. *Acta Oncologica* 2003;42:345–6.
23. Bouche O, Brixi-Benmansour H, Bertin A, Perceau G, Lagarde S. Trichomegaly of the eyelashes following treatment with cetuximab. *Ann Oncol* 2005;16:1711–2.
24. Pascual JC, Banuls J, Belinchon I, Blanes M, Massuti B. Trichomegaly following treatment with gefitinib (ZD1839). *Br J Dermatol* 2004;151:1111–2.
25. Chen AP et al. Grading dermatologic adverse events of cancer treatments: The Common Terminology Criteria for Adverse Events Version 4.0. *J Am Acad Dermatol* 2012;67:1025–39.
26. Hatch R, Rosenfield RL, Kim MH, Tredway D. Hirsutism: Implications, etiology, and management. *Am J Obstet Gynecol* 1981;140:815–30.

4

Photosensitivity and Photoreactions

Cecilia A. Larocca, Mackenzie Asel, and Mario E. Lacouture

Several cancer treatments provoke photosensitive eruptions. This skin toxicity is recognized by the Common Terminology Criteria for Adverse Events (CTCAE), created by the National Cancer Institute (NCI) for reporting in cancer clinical trials. Photosensitivity is defined as "a disorder characterized by an increase in sensitivity of the skin to light." In many cases, the mechanism of photosensitivity is not described, as it falls outside the scope of the clinical trial and it is not further defined by the CTCAE.

Classification of photoreaction type often relies on key clinical and histologic features described next (Table 4.1) (1–4). The most common mechanism of skin injury is a phototoxic reaction. Additional subtypes of photosensitive eruptions include photo-induced onycholysis, pseudoporphyria, and photoallergy (1). However, there may be significant overlap among eruptions. Additionally, drugs that induce phototoxic eruptions may also cause photoallergic eruptions. It is likely that other mechanisms of photosensitivity exist, as novel targeted agents and immunotherapies induce photosensitivity eruptions that challenge current concepts in photobiology. As such, in this chapter agents will be broadly referred to as photosensitizers when the mechanism of the eruption is unknown.

Treatment includes strict photoprotection, cool compresses, and in select cases where grade ≥2 severity is observed, topical and oral steroids may be warranted. Photosensitivity is not a contraindication to continuing therapy if symptoms can be adequately controlled with supportive care and strict photoprotection.

Phototoxic Reactions

Phototoxic reactions develop minutes to hours after ultraviolet (UV) exposure (1). Prior drug exposure for allergic sensitivity is not required. These reactions can occur in any individual and are dependent on drug dose, and intensity and duration of light exposure in the action spectrum of the photosensitizer (5). The action spectrum, specific to each chemical due to its molecular weight, is the range of wavelengths of light that, when absorbed, leads to an excited state. In the case of vemurafenib, the phototoxic eruption is triggered by UVA exposure (6). When returning to a lower energy state, energy is released in the form of heat, free radical formation, fluorescence, phosphorescence, or charge transfer, thereby causing tissue damage (5). Inflammation also plays a key role in the sunburn response. One such mediator is noncoding RNA, which after absorbing energy binds to toll-like receptors to trigger an inflammatory response (7). Additionally, certain cancer agents (e.g., taxanes) induce a phototoxic eruption by indirect generation of porphyrins (1,8,9). The clinical presentation in these cases (Figures 4.1 and 4.2) is indistinguishable from a classic phototoxic reaction; clinical and histologic features of porphyria are not seen. Alternatively, targeted therapies may cause an exaggerated sunburn-like response by interfering with the normal cellular response to UV-mediated injury (Table 4.2).

The clinical presentation and histologic appearance is that of a sunburn reaction, with confluent erythema in photoexposed sites (1). In severe cases, vesicles and bullae may develop within 24–48 hours after UV exposure. Over time, the skin may become tanned with sheetlike desquamation of scales. Photoexposed sites most commonly are the face and neck, with sparing of the nasolabial folds, folds of upper eyelids, deep furrows of face and neck, and those areas protected by the shadows of hair, ears and

TABLE 4.1

Features of Photoreactions

Photoreaction	Onset after UV	Prior Sensitization Required	Clinical Characteristics	Histology
Phototoxic	Minutes to hours	No	Exaggerated sunburn	Dyskeratotic and vacuolated keratinocytes, papillary dermal edema, endothelial cell activation, mixed neutrophilic and lymphocytic infiltrates
Photoallergic	Hours to days	Yes[a]	Acute, subacute, chronic dermatitis; eruption may spread beyond area of photoexposed sites	Spongiotic, possible interface or lichenoid inflammatory pattern[b]
Pseudoporphyria	Minutes to hours	No	Photobullous eruption with subsequent milia, scarring	Subepidermal bullae, sparse perivascular lymphocytic infiltrate, thickening of blood vessel walls
Hyperpigmentation	Minutes to days	No	Photodistributed hyperpigmentation with or without prior sunburn reaction	Melanophages with positive dermal Fontana stain and in some cases Perls stain
Photo-onycholysis	Days, (>14 days)	No	Distal splitting of nail plate	n/a
Photo-recall dermatitis	n/a	n/a	Sunburn-like reaction	Dyskeratotic and vacuolated keratinocytes

[a] Often on cancer treatment for several days prior to developing photoallergy.
[b] It is unknown if interface and/or lichenoid inflammation is unique to photoallergic reactions.

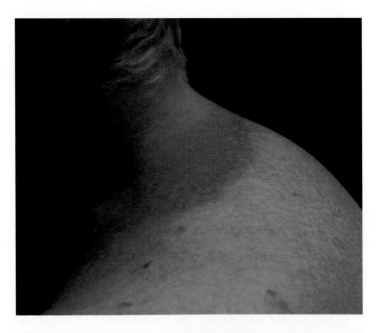

FIGURE 4.1 UVA-induced phototoxic eruption to vemurafenib. Patient with sharply demarcated diffuse erythema affecting only sun-exposed sites and sparing areas covered by her clothing.

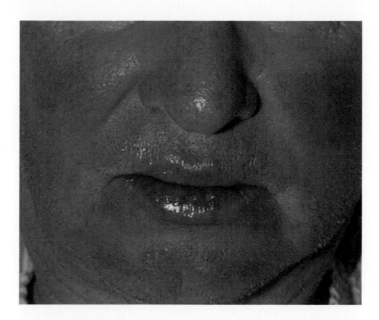

FIGURE 4.2 Vemurafenib-induced phototoxic eruption with erythema and vesicles in sun-exposed sites. (Republished with permission of John Wiley & Sons Inc., from Lacouture ME et al. *Oncologist* 2013;18:3.)

TABLE 4.2

Inducers of Phototoxic Reactions

Chemotherapy	Targeted Therapy
Dacarbazine	Dabrafenib
Dactinomycin	Imatinib
Doxorubicin	Lenalidomide
Fluorouracil	Vandetanib
Hydroxyurea	Vemurafenib
Mitomycin C	Retinoids (etretinate, isotretinoin)
Procarbazine	
Tegafur	
Thioguanine	
Vinblastine	
Capecitabine plus nab-paclitaxel	

Note: For further information, see References 6, 8, and 11–27.

nose. On the body there are sharp cutoffs between clothing and photoexposed skin, with erythema often restricted on the chest in a V-shaped distribution, extensor forearms, and dorsum of hands (1).

Treatment is supportive with use of soothing topical emollients. However, in the setting of extensive inflammation (edema, erythema, pain), topical and or oral steroids may be considered. Although photosensitivity is not a contraindication to continued treatment, for certain medications, such as dacarbazine, the severity of phototoxic reaction may worsen with continued exposure. Dose reduction and cessation of therapy have been needed in patients unable to follow strict photoprotection (10).

There are several variants of phototoxic eruptions (Tables 4.3 and 4.4) (1). Photo-recall dermatitis is the reemergence of a prior phototoxic eruption provoked by administration of drugs. In the case of methotrexate, photo-recall is induced if methotrexate is started days after ultraviolet exposure. As such, initiation of methotrexate may need to be delayed in patients who have had sunburn, phototherapy, or radiation therapy within the preceding week (28). It is unclear whether taxanes induce a true UV-recall

TABLE 4.3

Inducers of Phototoxic Reaction Variants

Chemotherapy	Targeted Therapy
Photo-onycholysis (8,11,29,30)	
Mercaptopurine	Vandetinib
Paclitaxel	Vemurafenib
Photo-recall (11,31–35)	
Gemcitabine	Sorafenib
Docetaxel	
Methotrexate	
Paclitaxel	
Pemetrexed	
Suramin	
Docetaxel–cyclophosphamide	
Etoposide–cyclophosphamide	
Methotrexate–cyclophosphamide–fluorouracil	
Hyperpigmentation (photodistributed) (11,36,37)	
Daunorubicin	Vandetanib
Doxorubicin	Vemurafenib
Fluorouracil	
Hydroxyurea	
Mithramycin	

dermatitis, given the similarity with another more common taxane-related toxicity: periarticular thenar erythema with onycholysis (PATEO), which, like a photoreaction, presents on the dorsum of the hands. Several cases of hyperpigmentation in photoexposed sites have developed (1,11). Hyperpigmentation may present immediately after sun exposure or as a delayed reaction after days of therapy without appreciable preexisting erythematous sunburn eruption. Photo-onycholysis is thought to be due to photosensitivity affecting the nail bed and develops 2 or more weeks after UV exposure (1,11).

Photoallergic Reactions

Photoallergic reactions require prior exposure for sensitization and thus often present after several days of therapy, often within 14 days of initiation (1,28). Clinically, these eruptions present as an eczematous dermatitis; spongiosis is seen on histology (1,5,28) (Figures 4.3 and 4.4). This is an uncommon skin toxicity from cancer therapies.

It is unclear if photodistributed eruptions with histologic appearance of erythema multiforme, interface, lichenoid or granulomatous dermatitis represent a true photoallergy or reflection of the cancer treatments' direct or indirect effect on the skin.

Photoexacerbated Disorders

Cancer therapies may cause dermatologic conditions that are exacerbated by exposure to ultraviolet radiation (Table 4.5). Chemotherapy, targeted therapies, and immunotherapy have all been reported to induce connective tissue diseases, such as subacute cutaneous lupus erythematosus, a photosensitive autoimmune condition (59–63). In particular, hydroxyurea has been associated with several photosensitive connective tissue diseases and is the most common trigger of drug-induced dermatomyositis (64–66). Tegafur has also caused dermatomyositis and lupus-like syndromes (11).

TABLE 4.4

Inducers of Photosensitive Eruptions[a]

Cancer Agent	Clinical Description	Onset[b]	Histology
Chemotherapy			
Epirubicin–bleomycin–vincristine (38)	Pruritus of sun-exposed legs within hours, erythematous edematous plaques that progressed to bullae at 48 hours at sites of scratching; positive photopatch test to epirubicin only	Day of first epirubicin infusion, bleomycin–vincristine ongoing therapy	Acanthosis, spongiosis, lymphochistiocytic infiltrate with eosinophils
Capecitabine (39–41)	Violaceous to erythematous, flat-topped papules or plaques with scaling on sun-exposed sites of trunk and extremities, one case with periungual erythema and scaling	2 weeks to 2 months	Interface dermatitis with lichenoid or basal vacuolar alteration, occasional necrotic keratinocytes, perivascular lymphocytes
Tegafur (42,43)	Erythematous lichen planus–like eruption in sun-exposed sites 24 hours after sun exposure; eczematous dermatitis in other reports	2 years	Interface dermatitis with perivascular mononuclear cells
nab-Paclitaxel (44,45)	Confluent erythema with scaling and hyperpigmentation with sharp cutoffs on sun-exposed sites of face, chest, forearms	1 month	Hyperkeratosis, mild acanthosis, spongiosis, sparse interface dermatitis and pigment incontinence
Hydroxyurea (46)	Pruritic erythematous macules, papules, plaques in sun-exposed sites	n/a	Noncaseating sarcoidal granulomas
Targeted Therapy			
Rovalpituzumab tesirine (47)	Photosensitivity, not further characterized in clinical trial; sunburn-like reaction within hours of sun (personal case)	1 week	n/a
Imatinib (48)	Sunburn-like; 3 months later developed lacy white striations of oral mucosa	1 year	Skin and mucosa with interface dermatitis
Sorafenib (49)	Photosensitivity, not further characterized in clinical trial		

(Continued)

TABLE 4.4 (*Continued*)

Inducers of Photosensitive Eruptions[a]

Cancer Agent	Clinical Description	Onset[b]	Histology
Vandetanib (37,50–54)	Pruritic lichenoid photodistributed dermatitis; three cases with painful or pruritic sunburn-like reaction with vesicles, erosions, and later with lichenified scaling plaques	1–24 weeks	Varying degrees of lichenoid lymphocytic infiltrate, spongiosis apoptotic keratinocytes
	Photodistributed target lesions of erythema multiforme; positive photopatch test	3 weeks	Vacuolar interface dermatitis, mild spongiosis, degenerated keratinocytes, perivascular and interstitial lymphocytes and eosinophils
	Pruritic near confluent erythematous eczematous plaques with vesiculation on sun-exposed sites 2 weeks after sun exposure	1 month	Superficial perivascular dermatitis with eosinophils and focal spongiosis
Flutamide (11,55)	Papulovesicular erythema or scaling of sun-exposed sites; one case progressed to erythroderma; some with positive photopatch test	2–5 months	n/a
Immunotherapy			
Nivolumab (56) Pembrolizumab (57) Ipilimumab (58)	Photosensitivity, no further description provided	n/a	n/a

^a Included are cases where the mechanism of photosensitivity is not described, photoallergic, or has overlapping features of photoallergy and phototoxicity.

^b Duration of cancer treatment prior to onset of skin eruption.

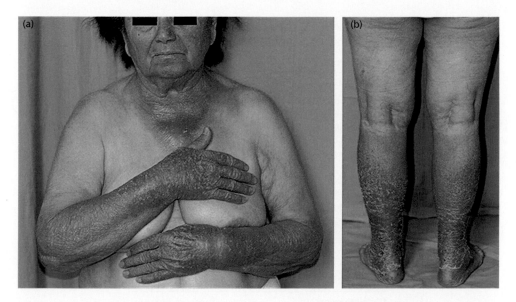

FIGURE 4.3 Vandetanib-induced photoallergic reaction. Erythematous edematous scaly lesions localized to the head and neck, décolleté, bilateral forearms (a) and legs (b). (Republished with permission of John Wiley & Sons Inc., from Fava P et al. *Dermatol Ther* 2010;23:5.)

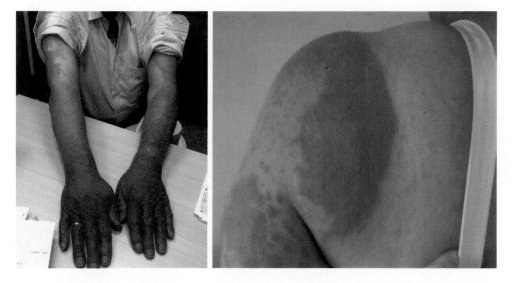

FIGURE 4.4 Vandetanib-induced photosensitive eruptions with varying morphology. (Reprinted by permission from Grande E et al. *Vandetanib in Advanced Medullary Thyroid Cancer: Review of Adverse Event Management Strategies*, Springer Nature: Springer Nature, Advances in Therapy, 2013.)

Epidermal growth factor receptor (EGFR) inhibitors cause cutaneous toxicity in a majority of patients and are well known for their association with a papulopustular eruption (Figure 4.5). Interestingly, the papulopustular eruption has been induced or exacerbated by UV radiation in some patients (67). EGFR inhibitor–induced rash often affects photodistributed areas including the face, upper back, and V of the chest. Interestingly, rash severity correlates with Fitzpatrick skin type; patients with type I to II skin have a 63% incidence of grade 3 or higher rash, as compared to 5% in skin types III to IV and 0% in skin types V to VI (10). This correlation may be related to the role of

TABLE 4.5

Inducers of Photoexacerbated Dermatoses

Chemotherapy	Other Therapies
Subacute Cutaneous Lupus Erythematosus	
Capcitabine (59,61,70,71)	Leuprolide (77)
Docetaxel (60)	Nivolumab (63)
Doxorubicin (72)	Tamoxifen (78)
Flurouracil (73)	Vandetinib (37)
Gemcitabine (62)	
Hydroxyurea (64)	
Mitotane (74)	
Paclitaxel (75)	
Doxorubicin–cyclophosphamide (72)	
Fluorouracil–capecitabine (76)	

Targeted Therapy
Acneiform Eruption
EGFR inhibitors (10)

Chemotherapy	Targeted Therapy
Porphyria	
Busulfan (11)	Flutamide (84–86)
Chlorambucil (79)	Imatinib (87,88)
Cisplatin (80)	
Cyclophosphamide (81)	
Fluorouracil (82)	
Methotrexate (83)	
Drug-Induced Pellagra	
Mercaptopurine (1)	
Fluorouracil (1)	

EGFR signaling in keratinocytes' protection against UV radiation–induced apoptosis and oxidative stress, which has been demonstrated *in vitro* (68,69).

Porphyria has been induced by several chemotherapies (3,11). Drug-induced porphyria is a photodistributed bullous disorder with clinical and histologic features of porphyria cutaneous tarda (vesicles, bullae, skin fragility, milia, and scarring) in the absence of the porphyrin abnormalities (3).

Pellagra, a photosensitive dermatitis caused by niacin deficiency, presents as an erythematous sunburn, followed by thickening of the skin, hyperpigmentation, and parchment paper–like scaling (5). It takes longer to recover from photoinjury compared to a normal sunburn. Select chemotherapies induce pellagra by interfering with niacin biosynthesis (1).

Photodistributed Disorders

Skin toxicities from cancer treatments that are photodistributed may be confused with photosensitive eruptions, but rather they reflect a prior history of photoinjury. A common example is inflammation of actinic keratoses (Figure 4.6 and Table 4.6). Erythema, pruritus, and increased hyperkeratosis within preexisting actinic keratosis usually presents within 1 week after initiation of chemotherapy (11). Additionally, lichenoid eruptions have been reported to a variety of cancer treatments. It is unclear if they are photoexacerbated or merely photodistributed. In cases of programmed cell death-1 (PD-1) inhibitor–induced lichenoid dermatitis, narrow band UVB has been used for treatment, arguing against an underlying photosensitivity (89).

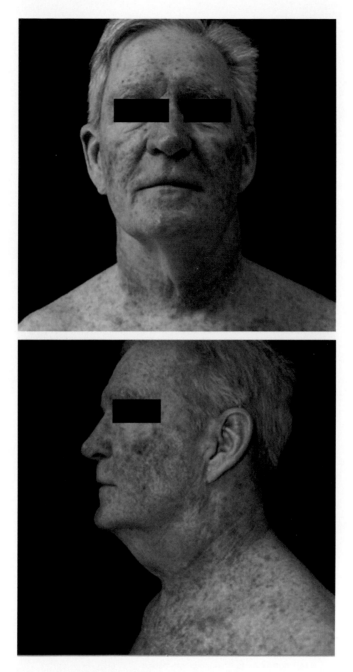

FIGURE 4.5 EGFR inhibitor–induced flare of acneiform eruption on photoexposed areas of face and neck. Note sparing skin under chin and sharp demarcation of erythema on the inferior neck at site of patient's shirt collar.

Conclusion

Chemotherapy, targeted therapies, and immunotherapy, regardless of the mechanism of action, can induce photosensitive eruptions. The most common cause of photosensitivity from cancer treatment is attributed to vemurafenib, with an incidence of more than 50% of patients (6,17,96,97). Aside from vemurafenib, vandetanib is also commonly associated with photosensitive eruptions, occurring in up

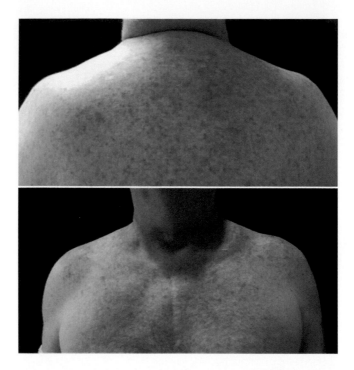

FIGURE 4.6 Photodistributed inflamed actinic keratosis. Patient with inflamed actinic keratosis located in predominately photoexposed areas of the upper chest and back.

TABLE 4.6

Inflammation of Actinic Keratoses

Chemotherapy	Other Therapies
Capecitabine	Erlotinib
Carboplatin	Sorafenib
Cisplatin	Sorafenib–tipifarnib
Dacarbazine	Nivolumab
Dactinomycin	Pembrolizumab
Deoxycoformycin	
Docetaxel	
Doxorubicin	
Fludarabine	
Fluorouracil	
Paclitaxel	
Pentostatin	
Vincristine	
Dactinomycin–darcarbazine–vincristine	
Doxorubicin–cytarabine–thioguanine	
Doxorubicin–vincristine	

Note: For further information, see References 11 and 90–95.

to 37% of patients (37,98,99). Interestingly, vandetanib has been shown to induce a number of different photosensitive eruptions, consistent with a phototoxic and photoallergic phenomenon. The varied clinical presentations include exaggerated sunburn, photodistributed lichenoid eruption, subacute cutaneous lupus with elevated antinuclear antibody, photoinduced erythema multiforme lesions with positive photopatch testing, photodistributed blue-gray pigmentation, and photo-onycholysis (13,15,30,36,37,50–53). Like vandetanib, fluorouracil is also capable of inducing a wide variety of photoreactions (1,3,11,73).

Early education about photoprotection prior to initiation of cancer treatment is critical in mitigating these reactions. In addition, given the long half-life of certain medications, it is wise to continue photoprotection even after discontinuing the offending agent. For grade 1 events, supportive care with topical steroids and antihistamines may be satisfactory. Systemic steroids may be necessary in grade ≥ 2 events. It is also important to recognize that patients may also be on other photosensitizing medications, such as antibiotics, diuretics, or nonsteroidal anti-inflammatory drugs (NSAIDs) (28).

REFERENCES

1. Gould JW, Mercurio MG, Elmets CA. Cutaneous photosensitivity diseases induced by exogenous agents. *J Am Acad Dermatol* 1995;33(4):551–73, quiz 74–76.
2. Gilchrest BA, Soter NA, Stoff JS, Mihm MC Jr. The human sunburn reaction: Histologic and biochemical studies. *J Am Acad Dermatol* 1981;5(4):411–22.
3. Green JJ, Manders SM. Pseudoporphyria. *J Am Acad Dermatol* 2001;44(1):100–8.
4. Rhodes LE et al. The sunburn response in human skin is characterized by sequential eicosanoid profiles that may mediate its early and late phases. *FASEB J* 2009;23(11):3947–56.
5. James WD, Elston DM, Berger TG, Andrews GC, editors. *Andrews' Diseases of the Skin: Clinical Dermatology.* London: Saunders/Elsevier; 2011.
6. Dummer R, Rinderknecht J, Goldinger SM. Ultraviolet A and photosensitivity during vemurafenib therapy. *N Engl J Med* 2012;366(5):480–1.
7. Bernard JJ et al. Ultraviolet radiation damages self noncoding RNA and is detected by TLR3. *Nat Med* 2012;18(8):1286–90.
8. Cohen AD et al. Cutaneous photosensitivity induced by paclitaxel and trastuzumab therapy associated with aberrations in the biosynthesis of porphyrins. *J Dermatolog Treat* 2005;16(1):19–21.
9. Akay BN, Unlu E, Buyukcelik A, Akyol A. Photosensitive rash in association with porphyrin biosynthesis possibly induced by docetaxel and trastuzumab therapy in a patient with metastatic breast carcinoma. *Jpn J Clin Oncol* 2010;40(10):989–91.
10. Lacouture ME, editor. *Dermatologic Principles and Practice in Oncology: Conditions of the Skin, Hair and Nails in Cancer Patients.* 1st ed. Hoboken, NJ: John Wiley & Sons; 2007.
11. Susser WS, Whitaker-Worth DL, Grant-Kels JM. Mucocutaneous reactions to chemotherapy. *J Am Acad Dermatol* 1999;40(3):367–98, quiz 399–400.
12. Scheithauer W et al. Phase II trial of capecitabine plus nab-paclitaxel in patients with metastatic pancreatic adenocarcinoma. *J Gastrointest Oncol* 2016;7(2):234–8.
13. Rosen AC, Wu S, Damse A, Sherman E, Lacouture ME. Risk of rash in cancer patients treated with vandetanib: Systematic review and meta-analysis. *J Clin Endocrinol Metab* 2012;97(4):1125–33.
14. Salvador A, Vedaldi D, Brun P, Dall'Acqua S. Vandetanib-induced phototoxicity in human keratinocytes NCTC-2544. *Toxicol In Vitro* 2014;28(5):803–11.
15. Son YM, Roh JY, Cho EK, Lee JR. Photosensitivity reactions to vandetanib: Redevelopment after sequential treatment with docetaxel. *Ann Dermatol* 2011;23(Suppl 3):S314–8.
16. Boudewijns S, Gerritsen WR, Koornstra RH. Case series: Indoor-photosensitivity caused by fluorescent lamps in patients treated with vemurafenib for metastatic melanoma. *BMC Cancer* 2014;14:967.
17. Boussemart L et al. Prospective study of cutaneous side-effects associated with the BRAF inhibitor vemurafenib: A study of 42 patients. *Ann Oncol* 2013;24(6):1691–7.
18. Brugiere C et al. Vemurafenib skin phototoxicity is indirectly linked to ultraviolet A minimal erythema dose decrease. *Br J Dermatol* 2014;171(6):1529–32.
19. Gabeff R et al. Phototoxicity of B-RAF inhibitors: Exclusively due to UVA radiation and rapidly regressive. *Eur J Dermatol* 2015;25(5):452–6.
20. Woods JA et al. The phototoxicity of vemurafenib: An investigation of clinical monochromator phototesting and *in vitro* phototoxicity testing. *J Photochem Photobiol B* 2015;151:233–8.
21. Carlos G et al. Cutaneous toxic effects of BRAF inhibitors alone and in combination with MEK inhibitors for metastatic melanoma. *JAMA Dermatol* 2015;151(10):1103–9.
22. Brouard M, Saurat JH. Cutaneous reactions to STI571. *N Engl J Med* 2001;345(8):618–9.
23. Liu W et al. The tyrosine kinase inhibitor imatinib mesylate enhances the efficacy of photodynamic therapy by inhibiting ABCG2. *Clin Cancer Res* 2007;13(8):2463–70.

24. Nardi G, Lhiaubet-Vallet V, Miranda MA. Photosensitization by imatinib. A photochemical and photobiological study of the drug and its substructures. *Chem Res Toxicol* 2014;27(11):1990–5.
25. Valeyrie L et al. Adverse cutaneous reactions to imatinib (STI571) in Philadelphia chromosome-positive leukemias: A prospective study of 54 patients. *J Am Acad Dermatol* 2003;48(2):201–6.
26. Perez-Paredes MG, Rodriguez-Prieto MA, Ruiz-Gonzalez I, Valladares-Narganes LM. Lenalidomide-induced photosensitivity. *Photodermatol Photoimmunol Photomed* 2013;29(6):334–6.
27. Ferguson J, Johnson BE. Retinoid associated phototoxicity and photosensitivity. *Pharmacol Ther* 1989;40(1):123–35.
28. Monteiro AF, Rato M, Martins C. Drug-induced photosensitivity: Photoallergic and phototoxic reactions. *Clin Dermatol* 2016;34(5):571–81.
29. Hussain S, Anderson DN, Salvatti ME, Adamson B, McManus M, Braverman AS. Onycholysis as a complication of systemic chemotherapy: Report of five cases associated with prolonged weekly paclitaxel therapy and review of the literature. *Cancer* 2000;88(10):2367–71.
30. Negulescu M et al. Development of photoonycholysis with vandetanib therapy. *Skin Appendage Disord* 2017;2(3–4):146–51.
31. Badger J, Kang S, Uzieblo A, Srinivas S. Double diagnosis in cancer patients and cutaneous reaction related to gemcitabine: CASE 3. Photo therapy recall with gemcitabine following ultraviolet B treatment. *J Clin Oncol* 2005;23(28):7224–5.
32. Droitcourt C, Le Ho H, Adamski H, Le Gall F, Dupuy A. Docetaxel-induced photo-recall phenomenon. *Photodermatol Photoimmunol Photomed* 2012;28(4):222–3.
33. Ee HL, Yosipovitch G. Photo recall phenomenon: An adverse reaction to taxanes. *Dermatology* 2003;207(2):196–8.
34. Basile FG, Creamer S. Docetaxel/cyclophosphamide-induced ultraviolet recall dermatitis. *Am J Clin Oncol* 2011;29(34):e840–1.
35. Magne N, Chargari C, Auberdiac P, Moncharmont C, Merrouche Y, Spano JP. Ultraviolet recall dermatitis reaction with sorafenib. *Invest New Drugs* 2011;29(5):1111–3.
36. Kong HH, Fine HA, Stern JB, Turner ML. Cutaneous pigmentation after photosensitivity induced by vandetanib therapy. *Arch Dermatol* 2009;145(8):923–5.
37. Giacchero D et al. A new spectrum of skin toxic effects associated with the multikinase inhibitor vandetanib. *Arch Dermatol* 2012;148(12):1418–20.
38. Balabanova MB. Photoprovoked erythematobullous eruption from farmorubicin. *Contact Dermatitis* 1994;30(5):303–4.
39. Hague JS, Ilchyshyn A. Lichenoid photosensitive eruption due to capecitabine chemotherapy for metastatic breast cancer. *Clin Exp Dermatol* 2007;32(1):102–3.
40. Walker G, Lane N, Parekh P. Photosensitive lichenoid drug eruption to capecitabine. *J Am Acad Dermatol* 2014;71(2):e52–3.
41. Willey A, Glusac EJ, Bolognia JL. Photoeruption in a patient treated with capecitabine (Xeloda) for metastatic breast cancer. *J Am Acad Dermatol* 2002;47(3):453.
42. Horio T, Yokoyama M. Tegaful photosensitivity—Lichenoid and eczematous types. *Photodermatol* 1986;3(3):192–3.
43. Usuki A, Funasaka Y, Oka M, Ichihashi M. Tegafur-induced photosensitivity—Evaluation of provocation by UVB irradiation. *Int J Dermatol* 1997;36(8):604–6.
44. Beutler BD, Cohen PR. Nab-paclitaxel-associated photosensitivity: Report in a woman with non-small cell lung cancer and review of taxane-related photodermatoses. *Dermatol Pract Concept* 2015;5(2):121–4.
45. Cohen PR. Photodistributed erythema multiforme: Paclitaxel-related, photosensitive conditions in patients with cancer. *J Drugs Dermatol* 2009;8(1):61–4.
46. Leon-Mateos A et al. Photo-induced granulomatous eruption by hydroxyurea. *J Eur Acad Dermatol Venereol* 2007;21(10):1428–9.
47. Rudin CM et al. Rovalpituzumab tesirine, a DLL3-targeted antibody-drug conjugate, in recurrent small-cell lung cancer: A first-in-human, first-in-class, open-label, phase 1 study. *Lancet Oncol* 2017; 18(1):42–51.
48. Brazzelli V et al. Photoinduced dermatitis and oral lichenoid reaction in a chronic myeloid leukemia patient treated with imatinib mesylate. *Photodermatol Photoimmunol Photomed* 2012;28(1):2–5.
49. Lam ET et al. Phase II clinical trial of sorafenib in metastatic medullary thyroid cancer. *Am J Clin Oncol* 2010;28(14):2323–30.

50. Caro-Gutierrez D, Floristan Muruzabal MU, Gomez de la Fuente E, Franco AP, Lopez Estebaranz JL. Photo-induced erythema multiforme associated with vandetanib administration. *J Am Acad Dermatol* 2014;71(4):e142–4.

51. Goldstein J, Patel AB, Curry JL, Subbiah V, Piha-Paul S. Photoallergic reaction in a patient receiving vandetanib for metastatic follicular thyroid carcinoma: A case report. *BMC Dermatol* 2015;15:2.

52. Bota J, Harvey V, Ferguson C, Hood A. A rare case of late-onset lichenoid photodermatitis after vandetanib therapy. *JAAD Case Rep* 2015;1(3):141–3.

53. Chang CH, Chang JW, Hui CY, Yang CH. Severe photosensitivity reaction to vandetanib. *Am J Clin Oncol* 2009;27(27):e114–5.

54. Fava P, Quaglino P, Fierro MT, Novelli M, Bernengo MG. Therapeutic hotline. A rare vandetanib-induced photo-allergic drug eruption. *Dermatol Ther* 2010;23(5):553–5.

55. Yokote R, Tokura Y, Igarashi N, Ishikawa O, Miyachi Y. Photosensitive drug eruption induced by flutamide. *Eur J Dermatol* 1998;8(6):427–9.

56. Robert C et al. Nivolumab in previously untreated melanoma without BRAF mutation. *N Engl J Med* 2015;372(4):320–30.

57. Sanlorenzo M et al. Pembrolizumab cutaneous adverse events and their association with disease progression. *JAMA Dermatol* 2015;151(11):1206–12.

58. Voskens CJ et al. The price of tumor control: An analysis of rare side effects of anti-CTLA-4 therapy in metastatic melanoma from the ipilimumab network. *PLoS One* 2013;8(1):e53745.

59. Ko JH, Hsieh CI, Chou CY, Wang KH. Capecitabine-induced subacute cutaneous lupus erythematosus: Report of a case with positive rechallenge test. *J Dermatol* 2013;40(11):939–40.

60. Chen M, Crowson AN, Woofter M, Luca MB, Magro CM. Docetaxel (taxotere) induced subacute cutaneous lupus erythematosus: Report of 4 cases. *J Rheumatol* 2004;31(4):818–20.

61. Fernandes NF, Rosenbach M, Elenitsas R, Kist JM. Subacute cutaneous lupus erythematosus associated with capecitabine monotherapy. *Arch Dermatol* 2009;145(3):340–1.

62. Wiznia LE, Subtil A, Choi JN. Subacute cutaneous lupus erythematosus induced by chemotherapy: Gemcitabine as a causative agent. *JAMA Dermatol* 2013;149(9):1071–5.

63. Liu RC, Sebaratnam DF, Jackett L, Kao S, Lowe PM. Subacute cutaneous lupus erythematosus induced by nivolumab. *Australas J Dermatol* 2017;59(2):e152–4.

64. Yanes DA, Mosser-Goldfarb JL. A cutaneous lupus erythematosus-like eruption induced by hydroxyurea. *Pediatr Dermatol* 2017;34(1):e30–1.

65. Seidler AM, Gottlieb AB. Dermatomyositis induced by drug therapy: A review of case reports. *J Am Acad Dermatol* 2008;59(5):872–80.

66. Layton AM, Cotterill JA, Tomlinson IW. Hydroxyurea-induced lupus erythematosus. *Br J Dermatol* 1994;130(5):687–8.

67. Luu M, Lai SE, Patel J, Guitart J, Lacouture ME. Photosensitive rash due to the epidermal growth factor receptor inhibitor erlotinib. *Photodermatol Photoimmunol Photomed* 2007;23(1):42–5.

68. Peus D, Vasa RA, Meves A, Beyerle A, Pittelkow MR. UVB-induced epidermal growth factor receptor phosphorylation is critical for downstream signaling and keratinocyte survival. *Photochem Photobiol* 2000;72(1):135–40.

69. El-Abaseri TB, Putta S, Hansen LA. Ultraviolet irradiation induces keratinocyte proliferation and epidermal hyperplasia through the activation of the epidermal growth factor receptor. *Carcinogenesis* 2006;27(2):225–31.

70. Floristan U et al. Subacute cutaneous lupus erythematosus induced by capecitabine. *Clin Exp Dermatol* 2009;34(7):e328–9.

71. Kim WI et al. Subacute cutaneous lupus erythematosus induced by capecitabine: 5-FU was innocent. *J Eur Acad Dermatol Venereol* 2016;30(11):e163–4.

72. Funke AA, Kulp-Shorten CL, Callen JP. Subacute cutaneous lupus erythematosus exacerbated or induced by chemotherapy. *Arch Dermatol* 2010;146(10):1113–6.

73. Almagro BM et al. Occurrence of subacute cutaneous lupus erythematosus after treatment with systemic fluorouracil. *Am J Clin Oncol* 2011;29(20):e613–5.

74. Mayor-Ibarguren A, Roldan-Puchalt MC, Gomez-Fernandez C, Albizuri-Prado F, Alvarez-Escola C. Subacute cutaneous lupus erythematosus induced by mitotane. *JAMA Dermatol* 2016;152(1):109–11.

75. Adachi A, Horikawa T. Paclitaxel-induced cutaneous lupus erythematosus in patients with serum anti-SSA/Ro antibody. *J Dermatol* 2007;34(7):473–6.

76. Weger W, Kranke B, Gerger A, Salmhofer W, Aberer E. Occurrence of subacute cutaneous lupus erythematosus after treatment with fluorouracil and capecitabine. *J Am Acad Dermatol* 2008;59(2 Suppl 1):S4–6.

77. Wiechert A, Tuting T, Bieber T, Haidl G, Wenzel J. Subacute cutaneous lupus erythematosus in a leuprorelin-treated patient with prostate carcinoma. *Br J Dermatol* 2008;159(1):231–3.

78. Fumal I, Danchin A, Cosserat F, Barbaud A, Schmutz JL. Subacute cutaneous lupus erythematosus associated with tamoxifen therapy: Two cases. *Dermatology* 2005;210(3):251–2.

79. Davies JH, Whitaker SJ. Chlorambucil and acute intermittent porphyria. *Clin Oncol (R Coll Radiol)* 2002;14(6):491–3.

80. Aramburo Gonzalez P, Roman Garcia FJ, Gonzalez Quintela A, Barbadillo Garcia de Velasco R. [A case of porphyria after treatment with cisplatin]. *Med Clin* 1986;87(17):738–9.

81. Manzione NC, Wolkoff AW, Sassa S. Development of porphyria cutanea tarda after treatment with cyclophosphamide. *Gastroenterology* 1988;95(4):1119–22.

82. Laidman PJ, Gebauer K, Trotter J. 5-Fluorouracil-induced pseudoporphyria. *Aust N Z J Med* 1992;22(4):385.

83. O'Neill T, Simpson J, Smyth SJ, Lovell C, Calin A. Porphyria cutanea tarda associated with methotrexate therapy. *Br J Rheumatol* 1993;32(5):411–2.

84. Schmutz JL, Barbaud A, Trechot P. [Flutamide and pseudoporphyria]. *Ann Dermatol Venereol* 1999;126(4):374.

85. Mantoux F, Bahadoran P, Perrin C, Bermon C, Lacour JP, Ortonne JP. [Flutamide-induced late cutaneous pseudoporphyria]. *Ann Dermatol Venereol* 1999;126(2):150–2.

86. Borroni G et al. Flutamide-induced pseudoporphyria. *Br J Dermatol* 1998;138(4):711–2.

87. Berghoff AT, English JC 3rd. Imatinib mesylate-induced pseudoporphyria. *J Am Acad Dermatol* 2010;63(1):e14–6.

88. Batrani M, Salhotra M, Kubba A, Agrawal M. Imatinib mesylate-induced pseudoporphyria in a patient with chronic myeloid leukemia. *Indian J Dermatol Venereol Leprol* 2016;82(6):727–9.

89. Shi VJ et al. Clinical and histologic features of lichenoid mucocutaneous eruptions due to anti-programmed cell death 1 and anti-programmed cell death ligand 1 immunotherapy. *JAMA Dermatol* 2016;152(10):1128–36.

90. Johnson TM, Rapini RP, Duvic M. Inflammation of actinic keratoses from systemic chemotherapy. *J Am Acad Dermatol* 1987;17(2 Pt 1):192–7.

91. Hermanns JF, Pierard GE, Quatresooz P. Erlotinib-responsive actinic keratoses. *Oncol Rep* 2007;18(3):581–4.

92. Lewis KG, Lewis MD, Robinson-Bostom L, Pan TD. Inflammation of actinic keratoses during capecitabine therapy. *Arch Dermatol* 2004;140(3):367–8.

93. Ali FR, Yiu ZZ, Fitzgerald D. Inflammation of actinic keratoses during paclitaxel chemotherapy. *BMJ Case Rep* 2015;2015.

94. Hardwick N, Murray A. Inflammation of actinic keratoses induced by cytotoxic drugs. *Br J Dermatol* 1986;114(5):639–40.

95. Lacouture ME et al. Inflammation of actinic keratoses subsequent to therapy with sorafenib, a multitargeted tyrosine-kinase inhibitor. *Clin Exp Dermatol* 2006;31(6):783–5.

96. Sanlorenzo M et al. Comparative profile of cutaneous adverse events: BRAF/MEK inhibitor combination therapy versus BRAF monotherapy in melanoma. *J Am Acad Dermatol* 2014;71(6):1102–9.e1.

97. Sosman JA et al. Survival in BRAF V600-mutant advanced melanoma treated with vemurafenib. *N Engl J Med* 2012;366(8):707–14.

98. Kharfan-Dabaja MA et al. Clinical practice recommendations on indication and timing of hematopoietic cell transplantation in mature T cell and NK/T cell lymphomas: An international collaborative effort on behalf of the guidelines committee of the American Society for Blood and Marrow Transplantation. *Biol Blood Marrow Transplant* 2017;23(11):1826–38.

99. Leboulleux S et al. Vandetanib in locally advanced or metastatic differentiated thyroid cancer: A randomised, double-blind, phase 2 trial. *Lancet Oncol* 2012;13(9):897–905.

5

Hyperkeratotic Reactions

Vincent Sibaud and Maria Vastarella

Secondary hyperkeratotic reactions have been frequently reported with systemic anticancer treatments. They are usually observed with tyrosine kinase inhibitors, but occurrence of hyperkeratotic lesions have been also described in association with cytotoxic chemotherapeutic agents and even with newly approved immune checkpoint inhibitors. Disruption of epidermal homeostasis and interaction with keratinocyte proliferation/differentiation or keratinocyte survival may lead to the development of a wide range of hyperkeratotic reactions, including hand-foot skin reaction, induced psoriasis, keratosis pilaris– or pityriasis rubra pilaris–like rashes, Grover's disease, contact hyperkeratosis, and squamoproliferative skin neoplasms (Table 5.1).

Hand-Foot Skin Reaction

Multikinase Angiogenesis Inhibitors

Hand-foot skin reaction (HFSR) represents the most frequent, dose-limiting, and clinically significant dermatological adverse event for patients treated with multikinase angiogenesis inhibitors targeting both vascular endothelial growth factor receptors (VEGFRs) and platelet-derived growth factor receptors (PDGFRs) (e.g., sorafenib, regorafenib, axitinib, cabozantinib, sunitinib, pazopanib). The overall incidence ranges from 5 to 60% (1–6), depending on the offending drug (Table 5.2). All-grade and high-grade rates are significantly higher with regorafenib, sorafenib, and cabozantinib.

Although it usually presents as a mild-to-moderate cutaneous reaction (grades 1 and 2), it may evolve into a more severe condition (grade 3) and represents the most likely cutaneous toxicity to result in treatment interruption or even treatment withdrawal. Moreover, although not life threatening, HFSR can lead to detriment in quality of life and can severely impair the patient's activities of daily living (7).

The presence of preexisting calluses and other hyperkeratotic areas, poorly fitting shoes, and repeated friction to the hands and feet represent well-individualized risk factors. HFSR is dose-dependent and more severe with higher doses. It has been also suggested that female patients, Asian patients, patients with specific genetic polymorphism, and patients treated for renal cell carcinoma tend to be more susceptible to develop HFSR (8). It may also represent a surrogate marker of clinical outcome (9), however, additional prospective data are needed.

Clinical Aspects

The clinical presentation is closely similar, whatever the inducing drug (2,9–13). HFSR usually emerges 1–5 weeks after therapy is initiated. It is characterized by tender, painful, bilaterally symmetrical erythematous and hyperkeratotic lesions on the palms and soles and on any areas subject to increased friction (Figure 5.1a through d). HFSR affects more frequently and severely the soles than the palms. Lesions appear and are predominantly located on pressure/friction points and on trauma-prone areas. They are classically distributed on the soles over weight-bearing sites such as heels, lateral aspects of the soles, and metatarsophalangeal/metatarsal skin areas. Palmar pressure-bearing surfaces such as the

TABLE 5.1

Main Hyperkeratotic Reactions Reported with Anticancer Therapies

Hyperkeratotic Reactions	Main Offending Drugs
Hand-foot skin reaction	Multikinase angiogenesis inhibitors (sorafenib, regorafenib, axitinib, sunitinib, cabozantinib ± pazopanib) Selective BRAF inhibitors[a] (vemurafenib, dabrafenib, encorafenib)
Psoriasis	Chemotherapeutic agents Angiogenesis inhibitors (bevacizumab, sunitinib, sorafenib) Anti-CD20 (rituximab) Bcr-Abl inhibitors (imatinib, nilotinib) Interferon alpha Immune checkpoint inhibitors (anti-PD-1, anti-CTLA-4)
Verrucal keratoses	Selective BRAF inhibitors[a]
Squamous cell carcinomas and keratoacanthomas	Selective BRAF inhibitors[a] Pan-RAF inhibitors (sorafenib, regorafenib) Immune checkpoint inhibitors (anti-PD-1) Chemotherapeutic agents (hydroxyurea, fludarabine)
Inflammation of actinic keratoses/ seborrheic keratoses	Chemotherapeutic agents (FU, capecitabine, taxanes, cisplatin, etc.) Selective BRAF inhibitors[a] Immune checkpoint inhibitors
Keratosis pilaris–like rash	Bcr-Abl inhibitors (dasatinib, nilotinib, ponatinib) Selective BRAF and pan RAF inhibitors
Pityriasis rubra pilaris–like rash	Ponatinib Sorafenib
Grover's disease	Selective BRAF inhibitors[a] Immune checkpoint inhibitors Chemotherapeutic agents, radiotherapy, endocrine agents
Others (cystic lesions, contact hyperkeratosis, verruca vulgaris)	Selective BRAF inhibitors[a] ± pan-RAF inhibitors

[a] In monotherapy. In combination with MEK inhibitors significantly restricts the development of hyperkeratotic lesions.

fingertips, thenar of the palms, interdigital web spaces, flexural surfaces of the digits, and skin overlying metacarpophalangeal/interphalangeal joints are also commonly involved.

HFSR generally starts with prodromal symptoms of tingling, burning, numbness, dysesthesia, or intolerance to contact. Then, well-demarcated painful yellowish hyperkeratotic patches ("callus-like hyperkeratosis") develop on friction and pressure-prone areas. A perilesional erythematous rim is frequently noted (Figure 5.1a through d). Large tense blisters and swelling can occasionally occur during the inflammatory phase. Patients may experience difficulty walking and holding objects. The resolution phase is characterized by an excessive desquamation.

TABLE 5.2

Hand-Foot Skin Reaction: Comparative Incidence Reported with Multikinase Angiogenesis Inhibitors (by Meta-Analysis)

Offending Drugs	All-Grade Incidence	High-Grade Incidence	Molecular Targets
Regorafenib	60.5%	20.4%	*VEGFR 1-3; PDGFR α-β; c-KIT; RAF; TIE-2; RET; P38 MAPK; FGFR-1*
Cabozantinib	35.3%	9.5%	*VEGFR 2; MET; RET; KIT; TIE-2; Flt3*
Sorafenib	33.8%	8.9%	*VEGFR 2, 3; PDGFR β; c-KIT; RET; RAF*
Axitinib	29.2%	9.6%	*VEGFR 1-3; PDGFR α-β; c-KIT*
Sunitinib	18.9%	5.5%	*VEGFR 1-3; PDGFR β; c-KIT; RET; Flt3; CSF-1R*
Pazopanib	4.5%	1.8%	*VEGFR 1-3; PDGFR α-β; c-KIT; RAF*

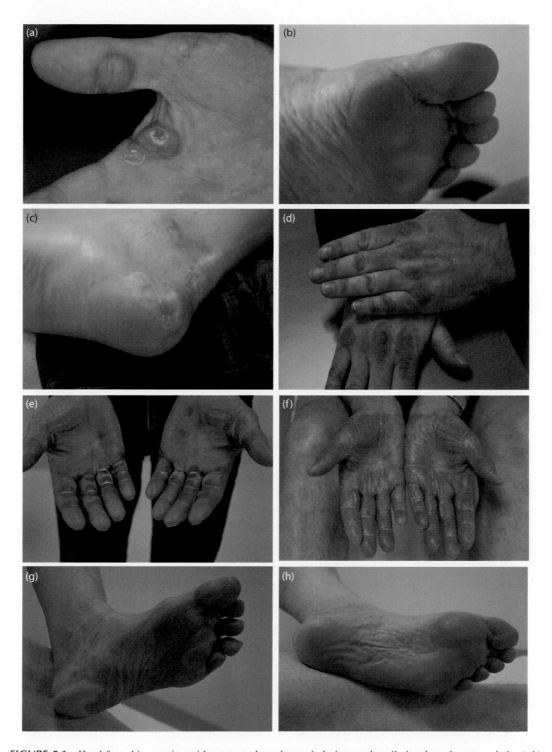

FIGURE 5.1 Hand-foot skin reaction with apparent hyperkeratotic lesions and perilesional erythematous halo. (a,b) Sunitinib, (c) regorafenib, and (d) cabozantinib (with visible lesions overlying the metacarpophalangeal and interphalangeal joints). (e) Grade 3 hand-foot skin reaction and (f) hand-foot syndrome induced by sorafenib and capecitabine, respectively. (Note major clinical differences: Hyperkeratotic lesions confined to friction areas versus a diffuse inflammatory erythema). Characteristic plantar callus–like thickening over pressure-bearing surfaces with BRAF inhibitors (g) encorafenib and (h) vemurafenib.

It is fundamental to note that HFSR clearly differs from chemotherapy-associated hand-foot syndrome, which usually manifests as a diffuse symmetrical palmoplantar and tender erythema that can blister and ulcerate (Figure 5.1e and f).

Histopathological Aspects

Histopathologic studies carried out in this context have remained relatively scarce (11,14). Skin biopsies revealed epidermal thickening with acanthosis, papillomatosis, parakeratosis, dispersed bandlike areas of dyskeratosis, and keratinocyte vacuolar degeneration. A mild perivascular lymphohistiocytic infiltrate is also noted into the dermis. The level of keratinocyte alteration is correlated with the time of exposure to the multikinase angiogenesis inhibitor.

Clinical presentation of HFSR is fairly typical and a skin biopsy should not be performed in this context.

Pathogenesis

The exact mechanisms of the pathogenesis of HFSR remains to be determined but are probably multifactorial. However, the development of HFSR appears to correlate with dose escalation of the multikinase inhibitor, which suggests that this may due to a direct mechanism-based effect. The development of similar lesions on other specific areas of friction (elbows, scars, dorsal aspect of metacarpophalangeal and interphalangeal joints; Figure 5.1d) may suggest that subclinical repeated microtraumas might promote the development of HFSR (15). Disruption of the repair mechanisms of endothelial cells, especially at the pressure and friction zones consequent to VEGFR inhibition may predispose patients to develop HFSR. VEGFR inhibition may be necessary but not sufficient to cause HFSR and that PDGFRs must also be inhibited. For instance vandetanib, which does not inhibit PDGFRs, infrequently results in HFSR. Conversely, it is unlikely that PDGFR inhibition alone accounts for HSFR, as the PDGFR-targeting agent imatinib mesilate does not cause HFSR. Similarly, bevacizumab, which specifically blocks the VEGF pathway, does not lead to HFSR. Consequently, dual inhibition of VEGFRs and PDGFRs could potentially prevent vascular repair mechanisms and could induce an inappropriate reparative response to ordinary injuries, thereby inducing HFSR in high friction/pressure areas (e.g., palms and soles) repeatedly exposed to subclinical trauma (11,12,15).

However, blockade of molecular-targeted VEGF/PDGF receptors would not be sufficient to explain all the molecular mechanisms of HFSR, as the incidence of HFSR from selective BRAF inhibitors is also high. It has been postulated that secretion of the multikinase angiogenesis inhibitor into the eccrine glands results in direct toxicity of the drug to the skin. No significant correlation, however, was observed between sweat secretion of sunitinib and sorafenib and the development or severity of HFSR (1,11). Moreover, no significant histopathological changes in eccrine glands have been individualized, making this theory unlikely.

Treatment

Appropriate education and counseling as well as preventive measures are required to reduce incidence and severity of HFSR (8,10,11,13,16). Avoidance of excessive pressure and repeated friction is the cornerstone of HFSR prevention. It is also critical to underline that the incidence and severity of HFSR is closely correlated to dose escalation and that transient dose modification or drug withholding leads to rapid improvement. Prompt identification and management of HFSR may be crucial to ensure proper dosing and to limit dose modification or treatment discontinuation.

Although evidence-based recommendations are lacking and management is mainly based on clinical experience and panels of experts, a step-by-step algorithm may be proposed (Table 5.3). Close monitoring is mandatory during the first weeks of treatment, and frequent communication between the treated patient and specialized health care professionals is required.

TABLE 5.3

Proposed Algorithm for HFSR Management (National Cancer Institute [NCI-CTCae], Version 4.03)

Grade 0/Grade 1—Minimal skin changes (e.g., erythema, swelling, or hyperkeratosis); without pain	**Patient education and preventive measures** Topical emollients twice a day Avoidance of traumatical activity, friction, excessive pressure or rubbing; reduce exposure to extreme temperatures Protection of pressure-sensitive or friction-prone areas Use of cotton gloves and socks, gel shoe inserts, padded insoles, shock absorbers, well-fitted shoes; avoid constrictive footwear; identify and remove prophylactically preexisting plantar callus/hyperkeratosis (address to podologist and/or use of topical salicylic acid 2–5% or urea ointment 10–50%)
Grade 2—Skin changes (e.g., blistering, bleeding, edema or hyperkeratosis) with pain; limiting instrumental activities of daily living	**Symptomatic management** Topical anesthesics (e.g., 2% lidocaine) and oral analgesics if needed High-potency topical corticosteroids (e.g., clobetasol) applied to affected areas Discuss celecoxib (100–200 mg/day) or oral corticosteroids **Continue TKI, reassess after 1–2 weeks and monitor for change in severity:** If worsened or intolerable grade 2, then decrease by one dose level, preventive measures (see grade 1) and reassess after 1–2 weeks; if improved to grade 0/1, discuss re-escalate dose; if worsened or intolerable grade 2 despite preventive measures, symptomatic management and dose reduction: manage as grade 3
Grade 3—Severe skin changes (e.g., blistering, bleeding, edema, or hyperkeratosis) with pain and limiting self-care activities of daily living	**Symptomatic management (see grade 2)** **TKI interruption, reassess after one week and monitor for change in severity:** If persistent or worsened, permanently discontinue TKI and supportive measures If improved to grade 0/1, do preventive measures (see grade 1) and resume TKI with decrease by one dose level, close follow-up, and discuss re-escalate dose If intolerable grade 2 or grade 3 despite symptomatic management, preventive measures and dose reduction, then discontinue

Abbreviation: TKI, tyrosine kinase inhibitor.

BRAF Inhibitors

Similar symptoms can be also observed in 20–60% of patients treated with selective BRAF inhibitors monotherapy (vemurafenib, dabrafenib) (Figure 5.1g and h) (17–20) that remain most often of low grade (grade 3 <2%) (21–23). Inflammatory palmoplantar hyperkeratosis seems to develop more frequently with the second-generation BRAF inhibitor encorafenib (24). Conversely, the overall incidence with the combination regimen containing BRAF and MEK inhibitors (cobimetinib, trametinib, binimetinib) is significantly lower (see section "Secondary Skin Neoplasms") (19,21–24). Of note, blisters are infrequently seen, and plantar surfaces are seldom involved. BRAF-related HFSR may persist for the duration of therapy (25).

Induced Psoriasis

Chemotherapeutic Agents

Complete or partial resolution of a preexisting psoriasis has been sporadically noted in patients treated with a wide range of chemotherapeutic agents with antiproliferative activity (26,27). Conversely, exacerbation of psoriatic lesions has been also reported with docetaxel (Figure 5.2a and b) (28). In our experience, however, both improvement and flares of psoriasis may occur with taxanes.

Targeted Therapies

Angiogenesis Inhibitors

By targeting VEGF (bevacizumab) or its receptors VEGFR 1–3 (sunitinib, sorafenib, pazopanib), angiogenesis inhibitors may improve psoriatic plaques in patients with a history of psoriasis (29–32).

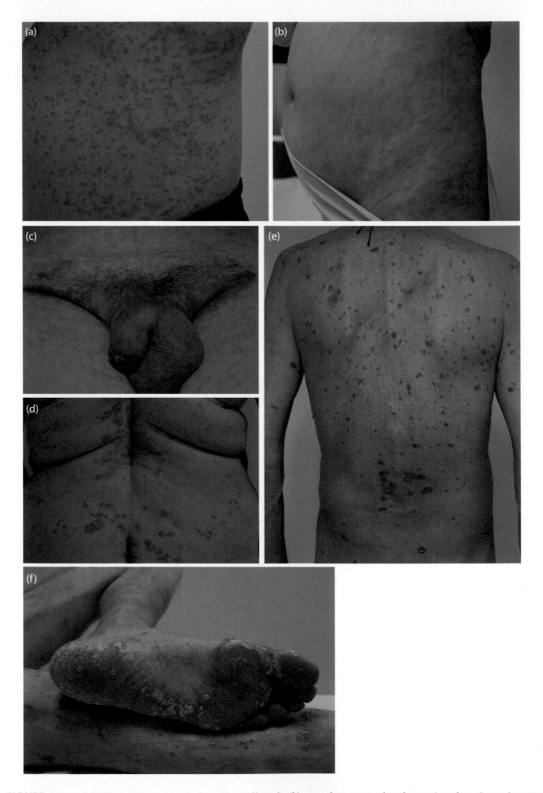

FIGURE 5.2   (a) Diffuse guttate psoriasis with paclitaxel; (b) complete regression 3 months after chemotherapy discontinuation. (c) Inverse psoriasis occurring with imatinib; (d) plaque psoriasis with idelalisib; (e) *de novo* psoriasis induced by anti-PD-1 nivolumab. (f) Plantar keratoderma associated with visible guttate psoriasis after anti-PD-1 therapy.

Moreover, the use of a topical sunitinib ointment in a specific mouse model was associated with alleviation of psoriasis-like inflammation, by regulating the keratinocyte proliferation and apoptosis (33). However, a paradoxical induction or exacerbation of a preexisting psoriasis has been also reported with both bevacizumab and multitargeted multikinase inhibitors (34,35).

EGFR Inhibitors

In the same way, treatment with epidermal growth factor receptor inhibitors (e.g., panitumumab, cetuximab, erlotinib) may also be associated with a rapid and prolonged improvement of concomitant psoriasis (31,36,37). It may be related to the direct inhibition of the EGFR signaling pathway, which is overexpressed in psoriatic keratinocytes. Psoriasis induced by anti-EGFR has been rarely noted (38).

Anti-CD20

Exacerbation or development of chronic plaque and arthritic psoriasis with rituximab has been individualized, although with a low incidence (39–41). Pathogenesis remains unclear. It could be hypothesized, however, that B-cell depletion may result in abnormal B-cell–mediated T-cell regulation.

BCR-ABL Inhibitors

Finally, BCR-ABL inhibitors (imatinib and to a lesser extent nilotinib) may also worsen or promote psoriasis (Figure 5.2c) (42,43). It is potentially related to a downregulation of regulatory T cells. We have also observed severe flares of plaque psoriasis in hematologic patients treated with the newly approved idelalisib and gilteritinib, which target PI3Kδ and Flt3, respectively (Figure 5.2d).

Anticancer Immunotherapy

Interferon

New onset or exacerbation of psoriasis is a well-identified adverse event of pegylated or nonpegylated interferon-alpha therapy. It mainly manifests as plaque-type psoriasis vulgaris. Topical management is often ineffective. Therefore, treatment interruption or systemic therapy is commonly required (44).

Immune Checkpoint Inhibitors

The risk of developing psoriasis with anti-PD-1/PD-L1 or anti-CTLA-4 agents is also well established (45–47), even though the actual incidence is currently unknown. Exacerbation or occurrence of psoriatic arthritis and even more skin psoriasis can be observed. Plaque psoriasis is the most frequent presentation, although guttate, pustular, scalp, palmoplantar, and inverse psoriasis have been reported (Figure 5.2e and f). The pathogenesis has yet to be defined. However, it has been previously demonstrated that the PD-1 pathway contributes to downregulate the Th1/Th17 signaling pathway (45). The management needs to be carried out in a multidisciplinary approach. In most cases, immunotherapy can be maintained and the patient managed by topical treatments (e.g., vitamin D analogues, topical corticosteroids). Acitretin and UVB therapy have also been administered in some cases as anti-TNF alpha therapy.

Secondary Skin Neoplasms

BRAF Inhibitors

Overview

One of the main drawbacks to highly selective inhibitors targeting specific activating mutations (V^{600}) of the proto-oncogene BRAF is the development of a spectrum of unanticipated cutaneous squamoproliferative lesions. It ranges from benign contact hyperkeratosis, hand-foot skin reaction (see section "Hand-Foot Skin

Reaction"), Grover's disease, or keratosis pilaris–like rashes to intermediate verrucal keratoses and malignant epithelial neoplasms (well-differentiated squamous cell carcinomas and keratoacanthomas) (17–20,25,48–50).

These BRAF inhibitor–induced hyperkeratotic lesions are thought to be the result of a paradoxical activation of the RAS-RAF-MEK-ERK (mitogen-activated protein kinase, MAPK) pathway in wild-type BRAF cells, leading to increased keratinocyte proliferation. Interestingly, the incidence of squamoproliferative toxic effects is significantly abrogated by the combination with a MEK inhibitor (either vemurafenib and cobimetinib, dabrafenib and trametinib, or encorafenib and binimetinib) (19,21–25,50,51). Concurrent inhibition with a MEK inhibitor of the MAPK pathway downstream may prevent this paradoxical activation, and consequently may reduce the development of secondary keratotic lesions.

Of note, the second-generation BRAF inhibitor encorafenib, with distinct pharmacological properties, may induce a lower paradoxical MAPK pathway activation in monotherapy (24). Finally, similar keratotic lesions can be also noted with pan-RAF inhibitors (sorafenib, regorafenib), also with a lower incidence (12,13).

Verrucal Keratoses

Verrucal keratoses develop between 21 and 79% of treated patients, and may represent the most frequent skin toxicity observed with single-agent BRAF inhibitors (17–19,21,23,48). No significant difference in gender is noted, but lesions are more common in older patients. They gradually occur in the first 3 months of treatment, but they can continue to appear throughout the treatment period (18,19,25,49). Conversely, they are clearly uncommon when patients are treated with a combination regimen with MEK inhibitors (19,21,23,25).

They present as white, wartlike, hyperkeratotic papules, which usually measure between 2 and 5 mm (18,19,25,49). They can develop at various anatomical sites, either with widespread distribution (in both photoexposed and nonphotoexposed skin) or with predominance on the head/neck and the trunk. Efflorescence of such lesions can be also seen (Figure 5.3) (20). Skin biopsy specimens reveal papillomatosis, acanthosis with hyperkeratosis, and mild to moderate epidermal dysplasia (17).

Because verrucal keratoses may present some degrees of dysplasia and may also represent a precursor of squamous cell carcinoma, destructive (e.g., cryotherapy, electrodessication), topical (e.g., ingenol mebutate, imiquimod), or surgical treatment is recommended. Moreover, lesions should be regularly monitored for changes indicative of evolution into squamous cell carcinoma. Lesions with a large size, a nodular aspect, a central keratin plug, a scaly ring, or a central ulceration should represent clinicomorphological features suggestive of a squamous cell carcinoma (SCC) in this context (52), and a skin biopsy should be performed for any atypical or suspicious lesion.

Development of new seborrheic keratoses and hyperkeratotic actinic keratoses have also been described (17).

Keratoacanthomas and Squamous Cell Carcinomas

Patients treated with vemurafenib/dabrafenib alone may also develop well-differentiated (Figure 5.4a through c) and keratoacanthoma-type (Figure 5.5a and b) cutaneous squamous cell carcinomas in

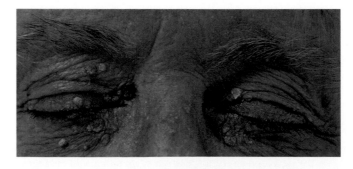

FIGURE 5.3 Efflorescence of verrucal keratoses with BRAF inhibitor in monotherapy.

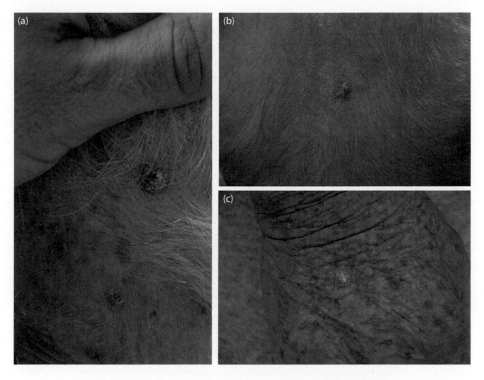

FIGURE 5.4 (a,b,c) Vemurafenib-related squamous cell carcinomas occurring on chronically sun-damaged areas.

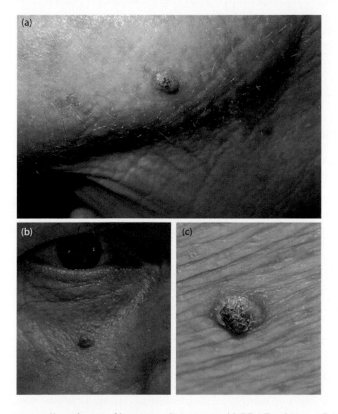

FIGURE 5.5 (a,b) Squamous cell carcinoma of keratoacanthoma-type with BRAF and (c) pan-RAF inhibitors.

approximately 20 to 30%, according to the series (17–22,50,51,53). The overall incidence is probably lower with encorafenib monotherapy (24). Secondary nonmelanoma skin neoplasms mainly occur in the first 3 months of therapy (17,20,49,52–54), although development of BRAF-induced SCCs has been also described after more than one year of continuous therapy (25). The perineal, genital, and oral mucosae can also be affected (18,55). A majority of patients generally develop one or two SCCs (20). However, eruptive lesions have been also reported (53,56).

SCCs/keratoacanthomas have been also described with pan-RAF inhibitors (sorafenib, regorafenib) (Figure 5.5c), but the incidence remains significantly lower (13,57). In addition, occurrence of SCCs in patients treated with BRAF and MEK inhibitors in a combination regimen is very unusual, with an overall incidence <5% (19,21–25,50).

The lesions are predominantly located on sun-damaged skin (head and face or limbs), but SCCs may occur in a variety of locations including non-ultraviolet (UV)-exposed areas (17,18,20,49,53,54). However, a background of solar elastosis and chronically sun-damaged skin is often individualized (20,48,58). Moreover, SCCs appear more frequently in older patients (>40 years old) and in patients presenting concomitant verrucal keratoses (17,25,49,53). Finally, a distinct mutational profile with a higher prevalence of activating *RAS* mutations (predominantly of the *HRAS* subtype) has been identified in epidermal neoplasms (i.e., verrucal keratoses and SCCs) arising in patients treated with anti-BRAF, preferentially in lesions developing in sun-damage skin (20,54,58–60). It has been postulated that the development of cutaneous SCC with BRAF inhibitor therapy is driven by a paradoxical increase in MAPK signaling, through the formation of RAF (homo/hetero)dimers (BRAF-CRAF, CRAF-CRAF) in wild-type BRAF keratinocytes with preexisting *RAS* mutations (54,58,61). By contrast, downstream inhibition of the MAPK pathway by concurrent inhibition of MEK leads to a significant reduction of skin tumor development (19,21–25,50,51). Finally, other contributing factors such as highly oncogenic human papilloma and polyomaviruses are unlikely to play a pivotal role in the development of BRAF-related verrucal keratosis or SCC (17,48,55,56), although available data remain conflicting (59,60).

The risk of metastasis is minimal in this context (53). Keratoacanthomas and squamous cell carcinomas, however, should be excised surgically with adequate margin borders. Chemopreventive measures such as systemic retinoids have been proposed in patients requiring regular or multiple surgical excisions for SCCs, and also for verrucal keratoses (62). Topical fluorouracil may be helpful. Dose adjustment or treatment interruption, however, is only exceptionally required (20). It is important to underscore an early detection, and patients require regular dermatologic follow-up throughout treatment with BRAF inhibitors monotherapy.

Chemotherapeutic Agents

Squamous Cell Carcinomas

It is now well established that long-term treatment with the antimetabolite hydroxyurea significantly increases the risk of development of actinic keratoses or basal/squamous cell carcinomas on photodistributed areas (63–65). Furthermore, lesions may appear abruptly after many months of treatment, with rapid growth and aggressive behavior (65). It has been demonstrated that hydroxyurea inhibits DNA repair in UV-exposed keratinocytes. Therefore, hydroxyurea may interfere with cell replication in the basal layers of the epidermis. Finally, the term "hydroxyurea-associated squamous dysplasia" has been proposed to individualize a precursor state associated with hydroxyurea, leading to the development of more aggressive squamous cell carcinomas (65). Detection of other hyperkeratotic lesions described in association with hydroxyurea is recommended (e.g., plantar/acral keratoderma, pseudo-dermatomyositis) (64).

Finally, fludarabine therapy may also represent a triggering factor for flare-up or accelerated growth of cutaneous squamous cell carcinomas (66).

Inflammation of Actinic Keratoses and Seborrheic Keratoses

The selective inflammation of subclinical or preexisting actinic keratoses and seborrheic keratoses may appear after exposure to systemic chemotherapeutic agents. This is particularly frequent with

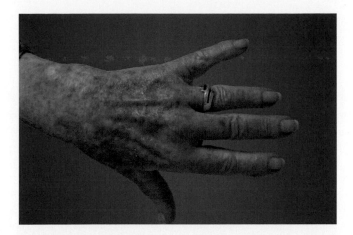

FIGURE 5.6   Inflammation of preexisting actinic keratoses on a photoexposed area with capecitabine.

fluorouracil and its prodrug capecitabine (Figure 5.6), but may also be observed with cisplatin, cytarabine, dacarbazine, dactinomycin, docetaxel, doxorubicin, and vincristine, either alone or in combination (28,67,68). It potentially results from the direct cytotoxic effect of chemotherapy on abnormal DNA synthesis in actinic keratoses.

Inflammatory, erythematous, pruritic, hyperkeratotic, scaly papules may develop on UV-exposed areas. The reaction is usually self-limiting and may even have a therapeutic benefit. Patient reassurance and supportive counseling is recommended. If the lesions are symptomatic, high-potency topical corticosteroids should be prescribed.

Immune Checkpoint Inhibitors

Eruptive keratoacanthomas and inflammation of actinic keratoses have been recently described with anti-PD-1 blockade therapy (69).

Cancer Survivors

The overall risk of subsequent neoplasms is significantly greater in cancer survivors. Nonmelanoma skin cancers represent one of the most commonly observed secondary malignancies, especially in patients treated in childhood or in patients treated with allogeneic hematopoietic stem cell transplantation (70,71). Radiotherapy, long-term treatment with immunosuppressive therapies, and graft-versus-host disease clearly represent well-individualized risk factors. It is therefore fundamental to ensure a continuous dermatologic follow-up for cancer survivors, with regular skin neoplasm screening.

Keratosis Pilaris– and Pityriasis Rubra Pilaris–Like Rashes

Bcr-Abl Inhibitors

Nilotinib and Dasatinib

Nilotinib and dasatinib are second-generation Bcr-Abl tyrosine kinase inhibitors that are approved for the treatment of imatinib-resistant (or -intolerant) chronic myeloid leukemia expressing the Bcr-Abl mutation.

The incidence of all-grade skin rash was evaluated by retrospective meta-analysis, and was about 34% and 23% with nilotinib and dasatinib, respectively (72). The most common presentation is a pruritic keratosis pilaris–like rash, which can involve the foreheads, cheeks, scalp, trunk, and proximal parts of the extremities (Figure 5.7a and b). Lesions usually start within 2 months of drug initiation, are

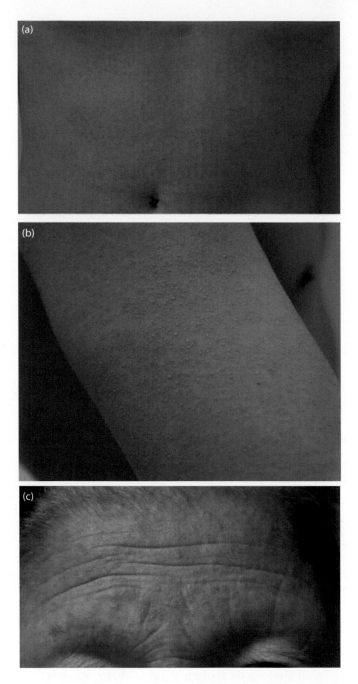

FIGURE 5.7   (a) Diffuse keratosis pilaris–like eruption with dasatinib, with (b) apparent tiny spicules. (c) Folliculocentric erythematous rash resulting from nilotinib therapy, with a characteristic grade 2 alopecia (eyebrows).

dose-dependent, and resolve after treatment discontinuation. Similar lesions, including perifollicular hyperkeratotic papules, hyperkeratotic spicules, and erythematous follicular–based papules, have been also described with nilotinib and dasatinib, which strongly suggests a follicular centric process (72–75). In this way, inflammatory nonscarring/scarring scalp alopecia with eyebrow involvement as well as body hair loss is frequently noted (Figure 5.7c) (73,75). It has been recently proposed that these lesions may be reminiscent of follicular lichen planopilaris (Graham-Little-Piccardi-Lassueur syndrome) (74).

The most prominent histopathological aspects combine perifollicular fibrosis, keratotic plugs within the follicle, follicular atrophy, and a sparse follicentric lymphocytic infiltrate (73–75). Pathogenesis remains to be elucidated. However, it could be related to a direct activity on several kinases (e.g., PDGF receptor, RAS/RAF, Src family), which potentially play a role in epidermal homeostasis (74,75). In addition, nilotinib and dasatinib may decrease TGFβ-stimulated collagen production (72).

Management includes topical corticosteroids, keratolytics (ammonium lactate, urea, salicylic acid), antihistamines, if needed. Due to the deleterious effect of pruritus, some patients may require dose reduction or temporary interruption.

Ponatinib

Ponatinib is a third-generation of Bcr-Abl inhibitor, which also targets fibroblast growth factor (FGF), PDGF, VEGF, FMS-like tyrosine kinase-3, KIT, and the Src families. It is now approved for drug-resistant chronic myeloid leukemia and Philadelphia-positive acute lymphocytic leukemia.

All-grade skin rash (not otherwise specified) is reported in about 35% of treated patients (74,76). In some cases, it corresponds to a fairly characteristic pityriasis rubra pilaris–like rash, which progressively develops 2 to 12 weeks after starting ponatinib (77–79). Lesions consist of well-demarcated pink-orange follicular-based papules coalescent into large pruritic plaques with powdery scales. Islands of sparing can be noted. They are predominantly located on the trunk, buttocks, thighs, and axillae with a bilateral distribution. Palmoplantar areas are usually spared. Histopathologic findings typically include a thickened cornified layer characterized by alternating of focal parakeratosis and compact orthokeratosis. A scant superficial lymphocyte infiltrate, mild spongiosis, and perifollicular fibrosis can be also noted (78,79). Management relies on keratolytics, topical corticosteroids, oral/topical retinoids, or UVB therapy, without requiring interruption of ponatinib.

A lamellar ichthyosis–like rash has been also described with ponatinib (78,80). Development of a folliculocentric exanthem with visible hyperkeratotic spicules and dyskeratosis, similar to those previously described with dasatinib and nilotinib, is also possible (74,78). Finally, patients can also present a combination of these dermatological changes.

RAF Inhibitors

A diffuse folliculocentric erythematous keratotic rash, mimicking a keratosis pilaris eruption, is also commonly observed in patients treated with exclusive BRAF inhibitors (18–20,50). It roughly affects more than one-third of patients (18,50). Lesions are mainly located on the trunk and extremities, with a sparing of the head and neck (18). Significant pruritus may be associated.

Similar lesions may occur more rarely with the pan-RAF inhibitor sorafenib (81) and, to a lesser extent, with regorafenib. In addition, a pityriasis rubra pilaris–like eruption has been exceptionally described with sorafenib (82).

Grover's Disease

Overview

Development of a transient acantolytic dermatosis has been described with a wide range of anticancer treatments. Grover's disease has been sporadically reported in patients treated with different chemotherapeutic regimen, radiotherapy, endocrine agents, or after hematopoietic stem cell transplantation (83,84). Immunosuppression may also represent a favoring factor.

It mainly manifests as a polymorphic, pruritic, erythematous, crusted papulovesicular eruption that is mainly located on the trunk and upper extremities. In this context, lesions may be more frequently extensive or atypical (83). Histopathological aspects include an epidermal acantholysis with different degrees of keratinocyte dysmaturation.

BRAF Inhibitors

Grover's disease is clearly more prevalent in association with selective BRAF inhibitors vemurafenib and dabrafenib prescribed in monotherapy. For instance, it has been individualized in up to 27% of patients receiving dabrafenib (17). It appears clinically and histologically indistinguishable from idiopathic Grover's disease, but lesions are only mildly pruritic (17). It can occur after more than one year of continuous therapy (25) but is not reported with anti-BRAF/MEK combination (19,25). It may be also related to a paradoxical activation of the MAP kinase pathway in normal keratinocytes (see section "Secondary Skin Neoplasms").

Immune Checkpoint Inhibitors

Finally, the occurrence of Grover's disease has also occasionally been reported with ipilimumab and PD-1 blockade therapy (45). The diagnosis is only confirmed after a skin biopsy, and its incidence is hence probably underestimated. A suprabasal acantholysis is isolated (Darier-like form), associated with a predominantly CD4+ T lymphocyte dermal infiltrate. Although rash and pruritus generally improve with topical corticosteroids, they can last for several months after treatment withdrawal.

Other Hyperkeratotic Reactions with BRAF Inhibitors

Contact Hyperkeratosis

Contact hyperkeratosis is almost exclusively observed with anti-BRAF therapy. It may arise over any site of chronic friction, in particular on nipples (Figure 5.8a). It may affect up to 12% of patients treated in monotherapy (18,19). Cheeks or even gingiva and buccal mucosa (Figure 5.8b) may be involved (55).

Verruca Vulgaris

Occurrence of verruca vulgaris (typically on digits) is also common with BRAF inhibitors (Figure 5.9a) (17,19,20,50). Viral inclusion with koilocytes has been individualized (25).

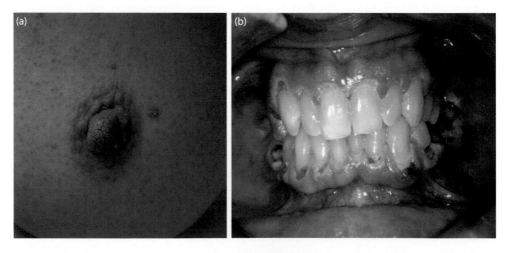

FIGURE 5.8 (a) Nipple hyperkeratosis and (b) mucosal hyperkeratosis involving the marginal gingiva with the single-agent vemurafenib.

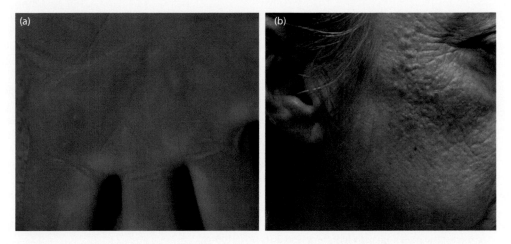

FIGURE 5.9   (a) Verruca vulgaris–like lesions and (b) milia with apparent facial cysts with the single-agent dabrafenib.

Cystic Lesions and Milia

Patients treated with selective BRAF and pan-RAF inhibitors can develop epidermoid cysts and milia (Figure 5.9b), which primarily involve the face (12,13,17,18,20,49).

REFERENCES

1. Belum VR, Wu S, Lacouture ME. Risk of hand-foot skin reaction with the novel multikinase inhibitor regorafenib: A meta-analysis. *Invest New Drugs* 2013;31:1078–86.
2. Belum VR, Serna-Tamayo C, Wu S, Lacouture ME. Incidence and risk of hand-foot skin reaction with cabozantinib, a novel multikinase inhibitor: A meta-analysis. *Clin Exp Dermatol* 2016;41:8–15.
3. Chu D, Lacouture ME, Weiner E, Wu S. Risk of hand-foot skin reaction with the multitargeted kinase inhibitor sunitinib in patients with renal cell and non-renal cell carcinoma: A meta-analysis. *Clin Genitourin Cancer* 2009;7:11–9.
4. Chu D, Lacouture ME, Fillos T, Wu S. Risk of hand-foot skin reaction with sorafenib: A systematic review and meta-analysis. *Acta Oncol* 2008;47:176–86.
5. Balagula Y, Wu S, Su X, Feldman DR, Lacouture ME. The risk of hand foot skin reaction to pazopanib, a novel multikinase inhibitor: A systematic review of literature and meta-analysis. *Invest New Drugs* 2012;30:1773–81.
6. Fischer A, Wu S, Ho AL, Lacouture ME. The risk of hand-foot skin reaction to axitinib, a novel VEGF inhibitor: A systematic review of literature and meta-analysis. *Invest New Drugs* 2013;31:787–97.
7. Sibaud V et al. HFS-14, a specific quality of life scale developed for patients suffering from hand-foot syndrome. *Oncologist* 2011;16:1469–78.
8. Chanprapaph K, Rutnin S, Vachiramon V. Multikinase inhibitor-induced hand-foot skin reaction: A review of clinical presentation, pathogenesis, and management. *Am J Clin Dermatol* 2016;17:387–402.
9. Wang P, Tan G, Zhu M, Li W, Zhai B, Sun X. Hand-foot skin reaction is a beneficial indicator of sorafenib therapy for patients with hepatocellular carcinoma: A systemic review and meta-analysis. *Expert Rev Gastroenterol Hepatol* 2018;12:1–8.
10. Zuo RC et al. Cutaneous adverse effects associated with the tyrosine-kinase inhibitor cabozantinib. *JAMA Dermatol* 2015;151:170–7.
11. Lacouture ME et al. Evolving strategies for the management of hand-foot skin reaction associated with the multitargeted kinase inhibitors sorafenib and sunitinib. *Oncologist* 2008;13:1001–11.
12. Lee WJ et al. Cutaneous adverse effects in patients treated with the multitargeted kinase inhibitors sorafenib and sunitinib. *Br J Dermatol* 2009;161:1045–51.

13. Robert C, Mateus C, Spatz A, Wechsler J, Escudier B. Dermatologic symptoms associated with the multikinase inhibitor sorafenib. *J Am Acad Dermatol* 2009;60:299–305.

14. Yang CH et al. Hand-foot skin reaction in patients treated with sorafenib: A clinicopathological study of cutaneous manifestations due to multitargeted kinase inhibitor therapy. *Br J Dermatol* 2008;158:592–6.

15. Sibaud V, Delord JP, Chevreau C. Sorafenib-induced hand-foot skin reaction: A Koebner phenomenon? *Target Oncol* 2009;4:307–10.

16. Anderson R, Jatoi A, Robert C, Wood LS, Keating KN, Lacouture ME. Search for evidence-based approaches for the prevention and palliation of hand-foot skin reaction (HFSR) caused by the multikinase inhibitors (MKIs). *Oncologist* 2009;14:291–302.

17. Anforth RM et al. Cutaneous manifestations of dabrafenib (GSK2118436): A selective inhibitor of mutant BRAF in patients with metastatic melanoma. *Br J Dermatol* 2012;167:1153–60.

18. Boussemart L et al. Prospective study of cutaneous side-effects associated with the BRAF inhibitor vemurafenib: A study of 42 patients. *Ann Oncol* 2013;24:1691–7.

19. Carlos G et al. Cutaneous toxic effects of BRAF inhibitors alone and in combination with MEK inhibitors for metastatic melanoma. *JAMA Dermatol* 2015;151:1103–9.

20. Lacouture ME et al. Analysis of dermatologic events in vemurafenib-treated patients with melanoma. *Oncologist* 2013;18:314–22.

21. Robert C et al. Improved overall survival in melanoma with combined dabrafenib and trametinib. *N Engl J Med* 2015;372:30–9.

22. Larkin J et al. Combined vemurafenib and cobimetinib in BRAF-mutated melanoma. *N Engl J Med* 2014;371:1867–76.

23. Long GV et al. Combined BRAF and MEK inhibition versus BRAF inhibition alone in melanoma. *N Engl J Med* 2014;371:1877–88.

24. Dummer R et al. Overall survival in patients with BRAF-mutant melanoma receiving encorafenib plus binimetinib versus vemurafenib or encorafenib (COLUMBUS): A multicentre, open-label, randomised, phase 3 trial. *Lancet Oncol* 2018;19:1315–27.

25. Anforth R, Carlos G, Clements A, Kefford R, Fernandez-Peñas P. Cutaneous adverse events in patients treated with BRAF inhibitor-based therapies for metastatic melanoma for longer than 52 weeks. *Br J Dermatol* 2015;172:239–43.

26. Cagiano R et al. Psoriasis disappearance after the first phase of an oncologic treatment: A serendipity case report. *Clin Ter* 2008;159:421–5.

27. Landi D, Santini D, Vincenzi B, La Cesa A, Dianzani C, Tonini G. Dramatic improvement of psoriasis with gemcitabine monotherapy. *Br J Dermatol* 2003;149:1306–7.

28. Sibaud V et al. Dermatological adverse events with taxane chemotherapy. *Eur J Dermatol* 2016;26:427–43.

29. Akman A, Yilmaz E, Mutlu H, Ozdogan M. Complete remission of psoriasis following bevacizumab therapy for colon cancer. *Clin Exp Dermatol* 2009;34:e202–4.

30. Narayanan S, Callis-Duffin K, Batten J, Agarwal N. Improvement of psoriasis during sunitinib therapy for renal cell carcinoma. *Am J Med Sci* 2010;339:580–1.

31. Overbeck TR, Griesinger F. Two cases of psoriasis responding to erlotinib: Time to revisiting inhibition of epidermal growth factor receptor in psoriasis therapy. *Dermatology* 2012;225:179–82.

32. Fournier C, Tisman G. Sorafenib-associated remission of psoriasis in hypernephroma: Case report. *Dermatol Online J* 2010;16:17.

33. Kuang YH et al. Topical sunitinib ointment alleviates psoriasis-like inflammation by inhibiting the proliferation and apoptosis of keratinocytes. *Eur J Pharmacol* 2018;824:57–63.

34. Yiu ZZ, Ali FR, Griffiths CE. Paradoxical exacerbation of chronic plaque psoriasis by sorafenib. *Clin Exp Dermatol* 2016;41:407–9.

35. Du-Thanh A, Girard C, Pageaux GP, Guillot B, Dereure O. Sorafenib-induced annular pustular psoriasis (Milian-Katchoura type). *Eur J Dermatol* 2013;23:900–1.

36. Oyama N, Kaneko F, Togashi A, Yamamoto T. A case of rapid improvement of severe psoriasis during molecular-targeted therapy using an epidermal growth factor receptor tyrosine kinase inhibitor for metastatic lung adenocarcinoma. *J Am Acad Dermatol* 2012;66:e251–3.

37. Goepel LM, Jacobi A, Augustin M, Radtke MA. Rapid improvement of psoriasis in a patient with lung cancer after treatment with erlotinib. *J Eur Acad Dermatol Venereol* 2018 February 11. doi: 10.1111/jdv.14862.

38. Mas-Vidal A, Coto-Segura P, Galache-Osuna C, Santos-Juanes J. Psoriasis induced by cetuximab: A paradoxical adverse effect. *Australas J Dermatol* 2011;52:56–8.
39. Guidelli GM, Fioravanti A, Rubegni P, Feci L. Induced psoriasis after rituximab therapy for rheumatoid arthritis: A case report and review of the literature. *Rheumatol Int* 2013;33:2927–30.
40. Mielke F, Schneider-Obermeyer J, Dörner T. Onset of psoriasis with psoriatic arthropathy during rituximab treatment of non-Hodgkin lymphoma. *Ann Rheum Dis* 2008;67:1056–7.
41. Thomas L et al. Incidence of new-onset and flare of preexisting psoriasis during rituximab therapy for rheumatoid arthritis: Data from the French AIR registry. *J Rheumatol* 2012;39:893–8.
42. Nagai T, Karakawa M, Komine M, Muroi K, Ohtsuki M, Ozawa K. Development of psoriasis in a patient with chronic myelogenous leukaemia during nilotinib treatment. *Eur J Haematol* 2013;91:270–2.
43. Shim JH et al. Exacerbation of psoriasis after imatinib mesylate treatment. *Ann Dermatol* 2016;28:409–11.
44. Afshar M, Martinez AD, Gallo RL, Hata TR. Induction and exacerbation of psoriasis with interferon-alpha therapy for hepatitis C: A review and analysis of 36 cases. *J Eur Acad Dermatol Venereol* 2013;27:771–8.
45. Sibaud V. Dermatologic reactions to immune checkpoint inhibitors: Skin toxicities and immunotherapy. *Am J Clin Dermatol* 2018;19:345–61.
46. Voudouri D et al. Anti-PD1/PDL1 induced psoriasis. *Curr Probl Cancer* 2017;41:407–12.
47. Bonigen J et al. Anti-PD1-induced psoriasis: A study of 21 patients. *J Eur Acad Dermatol Venereol* 2017;31:e254–7.
48. Chu EY et al. Diverse cutaneous side effects associated with BRAF inhibitor therapy: A clinicopathologic study. *J Am Acad Dermatol* 2012;67:1265–72.
49. Sinha R, Edmonds K, Newton-Bishop JA, Gore ME, Larkin J, Fearfield L. Cutaneous adverse events associated with vemurafenib in patients with metastatic melanoma: Practical advice on diagnosis, prevention and management of the main treatment-related skin toxicities. *Br J Dermatol*. 2012;167:987–94.
50. Sanlorenzo M et al. Comparative profile of cutaneous adverse events: BRAF/MEK inhibitor combination therapy versus BRAF monotherapy in melanoma. *J Am Acad Dermatol* 2014;71:1102–9.
51. Ascierto PA et al. Cobimetinib combined with vemurafenib in advanced BRAFV600-mutant melanoma (coBRIM): Updated efficacy results from a randomized, double-blind, phase 3 trial. *Lancet Oncol* 2016;17:1248–60.
52. Belum VR et al. Clinico-morphological features of BRAF inhibition-induced proliferative skin lesions in cancer patients. *Cancer* 2015;121:60–8.
53. Anforth R et al. Factors influencing the development of cutaneous squamous cell carcinoma in patients on BRAF inhibitor therapy. *J Am Acad Dermatol* 2015;72:809–15.
54. Su F et al. RAS mutations in cutaneous squamous-cell carcinomas in patients treated with BRAF inhibitors. *N Engl J Med* 2012;366:207–15.
55. Vigarios E et al. Oral squamous cell carcinoma and hyperkeratotic lesions with BRAF inhibitors. *Br J Dermatol* 2015;172:1680–2.
56. Dika E et al. Human papillomavirus evaluation of vemurafenib-induced skin epithelial tumors: A case series. *Br J Dermatol* 2015;172:540–2.
57. Arnault JP et al. Keratoacanthomas and squamous cell carcinomas in patients receiving sorafenib. *J Clin Oncol* 2009;27:e59–61.
58. Oberholzer PA et al. RAS mutations are associated with the development of cutaneous squamous cell tumors in patients treated with RAF inhibitors. *J Clin Oncol* 2012;30:316–21.
59. Frouin E et al. Cutaneous epithelial tumors induced by vemurafenib involve the MAPK and Pi3KCA pathways but not HPV nor HPyV viral infection. *PLoS One* 2014;9:e110478.
60. Schrama D et al. Presence of human polyomavirus 6 in mutation-specific BRAF inhibitor-induced epithelial proliferations. *JAMA Dermatol* 2014;150:1180–6.
61. Ali M, Anforth R, Senetiner F, Carlos G, Fernandez-Penas P. Mechanisms of BRAFi-induced hyperproliferative cutaneous conditions. *Exp Dermatol* 2016;25:394–5.
62. Anforth R, Blumetti TC, Clements A, Kefford R, Long GV, Fernandez-Peñas P. Systemic retinoids for the chemoprevention of cutaneous squamous cell carcinoma and verrucal keratosis in a cohort of patients on BRAF inhibitors. *Br J Dermatol* 2013;169:1310–3.
63. Antonioli E et al. Hydroxyurea-related toxicity in 3,411 patients with Ph'-negative MPN. *Am J Hematol* 2012;87:552–4.
64. Vassallo C et al. Muco-cutaneous changes during long-term therapy with hydroxyurea in chronic myeloid leukaemia. *Clin Exp Dermatol* 2001;26:141–8.

65. Sanchez-Palacios C, Guitart J. Hydroxyurea-associated squamous dysplasia. *J Am Acad Dermatol* 2004;51:293–300.
66. Herr D, Borelli S, Kempf W, Trojan A. Fludarabine: Risk factor for aggressive behaviour of squamous cell carcinoma of the skin? *Ann Oncol* 2005;16:515–6.
67. Peramiquel L, Dalmau J, Puig L, Roé E, Fernández-Figueras MT, Alomar A. Inflammation of actinic keratoses and acral erythrodysesthesia during capecitabine treatment. *J Am Acad Dermatol* 2006;55:S119–20.
68. Johnson TM, Rapini RP, Duvic M. Inflammation of actinic keratoses from systemic chemotherapy. *J Am Acad Dermatol* 1987;17:192–7.
69. Freites-Martinez A, Kwong BY, Rieger KE, Coit DG, Colevas AD, Lacouture ME. Eruptive keratoacanthomas associated with pembrolizumab therapy. *JAMA Dermatol* 2017;153:694–7.
70. Turcotte LM et al. Risk of subsequent neoplasms during the fifth and sixth decades of life in the childhood cancer survivor study cohort. *J Clin Oncol* 2015;33:3568–75.
71. Leisenring W, Friedman DL, Flowers MED, Schwartz JL, Deeg HJ. Nonmelanoma skin and mucosal cancers after hematopoietic cell transplantation. *J Clin Oncol* 2006;24:1119–24.
72. Drucker AM, Wu S, Busam KJ, Berman E, Amitay-Laish I, Lacouture ME. Rash with the multitargeted kinase inhibitors nilotinib and dasatinib: Meta-analysis and clinical characterization. *Eur J Haematol* 2013;90:142–50.
73. Delgado L et al. Adverse cutaneous reactions to the new second-generation tyrosine kinase inhibitors (dasatinib, nilotinib) in chronic myeloid leukemia. *J Am Acad Dermatol* 2013;69:839–40.
74. Patel AB, Solomon AR, Mauro MJ, Ehst BD. Unique cutaneous reaction to second- and third-generation tyrosine kinase inhibitors for chronic myeloid leukemia. *Dermatology* 2016;232:122–5.
75. Hansen T, Little AJ, Miller JJ, Ioffreda MD. A case of inflammatory nonscarring alopecia associated with the tyrosine kinase inhibitor nilotinib. *JAMA Dermatol* 2013;149:330–2.
76. Cortes JE et al. A phase 2 trial of ponatinib in Philadelphia chromosome-positive leukemias. *N Engl J Med* 2013;369:1783–96.
77. Jack A, Mauro MJ, Ehst BD. Pityriasis rubra pilaris–like eruption associated with the multikinase inhibitor ponatinib. *J Am Acad Dermatol* 2013;69:249–50.
78. Alloo A et al. Ponatinib-induced pityriasiform, folliculocentric and ichthyosiform cutaneous toxicities. *Br J Dermatol* 2015;173:574–7.
79. Eber AE, Rosen A, Oberlin KE, Giubellino A, Romanelli P. Ichthyosiform pityriasis rubra pilaris-like eruption secondary to ponatinib therapy: Case report and literature review. *Drug Saf Case Rep* 2017;4:19.
80. Örenay ÖM, Tamer F, Sarıfakıoğlu E, Yıldırım U. Lamellar ichthyosis-like eruption associated with ponatinib. *Acta Dermatovenerol Alp Pannonica Adriat* 2016;25:59–60.
81. Kong HH, Turner ML. Array of cutaneous adverse effects associated with sorafenib. *J Am Acad Dermatol* 2009;61:360–1.
82. Paz C, Querfeld C, Shea CR. Sorafenib-induced eruption resembling pityriasis rubra pilaris. *J Am Acad Dermatol* 2011;65:452–3.
83. Gantz M, Butler D, Goldberg M, Ryu J, McCalmont T, Shinkai K. Atypical features and systemic associations in extensive cases of Grover disease: A systematic review. *J Am Acad Dermatol* 2017;77:952–7.
84. Villalon G, Martin JM, Monteagudo C, Alonso V, Ramon D, Jorda E. Clinicopathological spectrum of chemotherapy induced Grover's disease. *J Eur Acad Dermatol Venereol* 2007;21:1145–7.

6

Sclerotic Eruptions

Bernice Y. Kwong

Sclerotic reactions can develop during treatment with various cancer therapies. These reactions are rare and range in presentation from localized hardening of the skin to possible induction or worsening of autoimmune connective tissue disease such as systemic sclerosis (scleroderma). These reactions are thought to be due to chemotherapy-induced accumulation of extracellular matrix proteins into the skin, possibly mediated by TGF-beta. Clinical manifestations of sclerotic reactions induced by cancer therapy can be varied and include atrophic white, shiny sclerotic plaques (lichen sclerosus et atrophicus), inflammatory induration and thickening of the dermal layer of the skin (morphea/localized scleroderma), sclerosis of the lower legs with an "inverted champagne bottle" appearance (lipodermatosclerosis), or tender edematous warm plaques that mimic cellulitis (pseudocellulitis). Patients with a history of underlying systemic sclerosis may experience worsening of underlying induration, edema, or even ulceration. Rarely, some anticancer agents have been reported to be associated with *de novo* autoantibody-positive systemic sclerosis.

Bleomycin-Induced Acrosclerosis

The antitumor antibiotic bleomycin is associated with sclerosis of the lung and skin (1–3). Cutaneous sclerosis is thought to be dependent on cumulative dose and has been reported at cumulative doses of bleomycin ranging from 51 to 780 IU. There is a possible male predominance and increased risk in patients with renal dysfunction due to excretion of the drug through the kidney (4).

Bleomycin-induced sclerotic reactions in the skin most commonly involve the hands and feet in an "acrosclerosis" distribution, sparing the trunk and face. The reaction starts as edematous plaques on the hands, forearms, and feet that develop several months after drug initiation and subsequently evolve over the course of months to hyperpigmented indurated plaques overlying the fingers and joints. Sclerotic bands on the fingers may impede function, and digital ulcerations can develop. On skin biopsy, homogenized collagen is seen in the dermis around blood vessels and adnexal structures (2). Although features of systemic sclerosis such as telangiectasias, periungual erythema, calcinosis cutis, and autoantibodies are usually absent, pulmonary fibrosis may accompany the cutaneous sclerotic changes.

The pathogenesis of bleomycin-induced sclerosis is unknown, however, it is thought to be due to direct toxicity by lipid peroxidation and DNA stand breakage. Bleomycin hydrolase—the enzyme responsible for inactivating bleomycin—is deficient in both the skin and in the lungs, correlating with the organs that have the most toxicity from the drug (5,6). Bleomycin injection into murine skin leads to the development of a scleroderma-like dermal sclerosis with accompanying sclerotic lung changes in the mice, with higher concentrations of the drug found in the skin and lungs, likely attributing to local toxicity to these two organs. Biopsy of sclerotic skin in affected mice show increased dermal thickness, thickened collagen fibers and deposition, thickened vascular wall, increased mast cells, and increased procollagen gene expression as well as transforming growth factor-beta (TGF-beta) and C-C motif chemokine ligand 2 (CCL2) expression.

Treatment of bleomycin-induced acrosclerosis can be difficult and may include nifedipine, nicotinamide, and aspirin. Bevacizumab can prevent bleomycin-induced dermal fibrosis in the mouse model (7). In most patients, sclerosis will improve after bleomycin is discontinued, however, sclerotic changes over distal phalanges have been described to persist (8).

Taxane Therapy–Related Sclerodermatous Dermatitis

The antimicrotubule agents paclitaxel and docetaxel are rarely associated with scleroderma-like reactions in the skin at total cumulative doses ranging from 300 to 2625 mg/m² (9). Edema occurs in 47% of patients receiving taxane therapy, and in some of these cases, this initial inflammatory edema (Figure 6.1) eventually leads to sclerosis and hyperpigmentation, most commonly involving the extremities with a predilection for the lower extremities. The initial edema may start 6 months to several years after treatment initiation and may precede sclerosis by 5–12 months (10,11). Involvement over the joints may lead to contractures. There appears to be a female predominance, however, this may be due to the high frequency of taxane use in breast and ovarian cancers, which occur more in females. Taxane therapy–induced cutaneous sclerosis has been reported to worsen after one single dose of carboplatin (12).

Although the clinical presentation of taxane-induced sclerosis of the extremities can mimic systemic sclerosis, there are usually no cuticular changes or telangiectasias, and autoantibodies are not detected. A unique clinical feature of taxane-induced cutaneous sclerosis that may help distinguish it from systemic sclerosis is a predilection of the sclerosis to present as proximal extremity sclerosis—the induration tends to be more pronounced at the calf and ankle compared to more distal sclerosis, leaving the distal foot spared (Figure 6.2) (11).

There are rare reports of autoimmune antibody-negative systemic sclerosis, with widespread sclerosis and internal organ involvement, including myocarditis, secondary to paclitaxel (13). Rarely, have patients been reported to develop a positive antinuclear antibody (ANA) with a discrete, speckled pattern; and there has been one case with positive anticentromere antibodies (10).

On histopathologic examination, findings from skin biopsy in patients with taxane-related cutaneous sclerosis are identical to those seen in systemic sclerosis. The pathophysiology is unclear and may be due to activation of tumor necrosis factor-alpha (TNF-alpha), interleukin-2, and interleukin-6, as well as various cytokines that stimulate fibroblast proliferation.

Treatments for taxane-induced sclerosis include topical and systemic steroids, physical therapy, and systemic methotrexate. In general, edema improves and skin ultimately softens after drug discontinuation; however, there may be persistent hidebound hardening of the skin even after drug discontinuation (Figure 6.3).

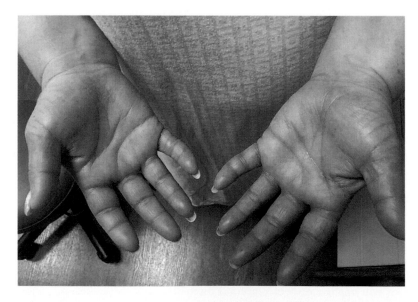

FIGURE 6.1   Inflammatory edema in a patient on taxane therapy, leading to sclerosis and hyperpigmentation.

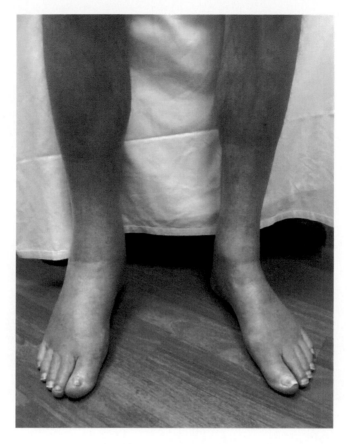

FIGURE 6.2 Proximal extremity sclerosis in a patient on taxane therapy.

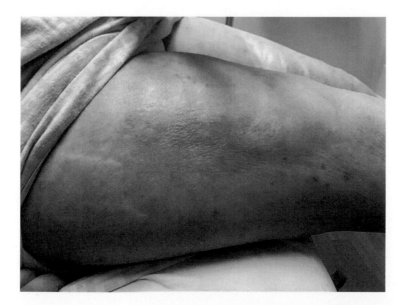

FIGURE 6.3 Persistent hidebound hardening of the skin even after the patient had discontinued taxane therapy.

Antimetabolite-Related Cutaneous Sclerosis of the Extremities

5-Fluorouracil, Capecitabine, Uracil–Tegafur

Hand-foot syndrome (HFS), also called palmoplantar erythrodysesthesia, is the most common adverse event arising during treatment with 5-fluorouracil or its prodrugs capecitabine or uracil–tegafur (UFT), and up to 68% of patients receiving capecitabine develop HFS by the end of the second cycle (14). Rarely, patients may develop a more severe, sclerotic form of HFS reaction that presents with painful, waxy, shiny erythema and edema, accompanied by eventual sclerosis, keratoderma-like thickening of the skin, and occasionally sclerodactyly of the hands and fingers (Figure 6.4) (15–18). In darker skin types, the first signs of this sclerotic form of HFS can be hyperpigmentation (Figure 6.5) (19).

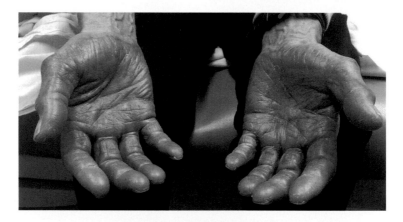

FIGURE 6.4   Severe, sclerotic form of HFS reaction in a patient on 5-fluorouracil therapy.

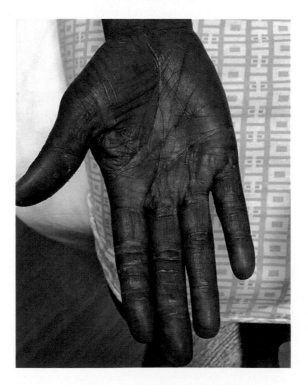

FIGURE 6.5   Stiff, keratoderma-like thickening of the skin in a patient on 5-fluorouracil therapy.

Skin biopsy from patients with sclerotic HFS changes during capecitabine therapy shows sclerosis of the papillary and reticular dermis, with thick homogeneous eosinophilic collagen bundles, which is not seen in typical or classic HFS (15). Treatment includes supportive measures such as topical steroids, emolliation, elevation, cold compresses, and topical anesthetics. Systemic corticosteroids (e.g., celecoxib, 200 mg PO twice daily for 14 days per cycle in patients without history of cardiovascular disease) may be helpful. In severe cases, dose reduction or interruption of therapy may be necessary (20).

Pemetrexed

During treatment of cancer with the antifolate compound pemetrexed, peripheral edema is common, affecting approximately 13% of patients (21). Like with other antimetabolite agents, a subset of these patients will develop an inflammatory edema, which subsequently progresses into sclerosis over the extremities accompanied by hyperpigmentation. This reaction has also been described as lipodermatosclerosis, "sclerosing panniculitis," or "pseudocellulitis." Patients present with initial painful erythema, warmth, and tenderness on the extremities representing inflammation of the subcutaneous fat, which can clinically be mistaken for cellulitis (Figure 6.6), and later develop hardened, hyperpigmented bound-down sclerotic skin with an inverse champagne bottle appearance. The severity of cutaneous toxicity increases with number of cycles of pemetrexed received, and there is a possible female predominance. Skin biopsies from the scleroderma-like eruptions show thickening of the dermis with perivascular lymphocytes.

This reaction is possibly associated with fluid retention and therefore there may be an increased risk in patients with history of lower extremity edema due to lymphedema or stasis dermatitis or deep vein thrombosis. In addition, patients who have history of receiving other antimetabolite drugs such as gemcitabine, may have an increased risk.

Treatment includes topical steroids, emolliation, elevation, and compression stockings for edema (22). Prophylactic treatment with systemic corticosteroids (oral dexamethasone 4 mg by mouth twice daily or prednisolone 50 mg daily starting the day prior to treatment for 3 days total) can lead to decreased severity of cutaneous toxicities (23).

Gemcitabine

Peripheral edema is common during treatment with the nucleoside analog gemcitabine, occurring in approximately 20.3% of patients (24). This cutaneous reaction has been termed pseudocellulitis, lipodermatosclerosis-like, or a scleroderma-like reaction (25). In these cases, the inflammatory edema presents as painful edematous red plaques, usually restricted to the lower extremities, sparing the feet

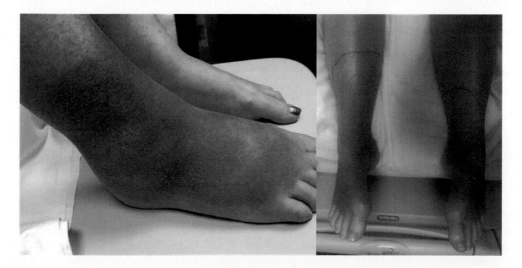

FIGURE 6.6 Inflammation of the subcutaneous fat in a patient on pemetrexed therapy.

and starting above the ankles. The initial edema then gives way to more sclerodermatous changes including hide-bound indurated skin with accompanying hyperpigmentation. There may be associated difficulty with extension/flexion. The clinical picture may be misinterpreted as cellulitis or deep vein thrombosis.

The mechanism of sclerotic skin changes due to gemcitabine is unclear but is theorized to be secondary to accumulation of drug into the subcutaneous tissues. Prior to starting gemcitabine therapy, patients who have underlying stasis dermatitis or lymphedema should be counseled to take precautionary interventions. Patients with history of systemic sclerosis receiving carboplatin and gemcitabine may be at increased risk of worsening of their lesions, leading to digital necrosis (26).

Treatment options include high-potency topical steroids under occlusion, elevation, compression garments, or low-dose systemic steroids. Softening usually improves over time if the drug is discontinued.

Hydroxyurea

Hydroxyurea has been reported to cause painful edema on the legs, which can lead to woody induration of the skin with negative autoantibodies. In one case, indurated lesions resolved after hydroxyurea was switched to anagrelide (27).

Scleroderma-Like Reactions to Other Agents

Scleroderma-like tightening of the skin in the absence of positive autoantibodies has also been reported with several other chemotherapeutic agents, including localized scleroderma developing in patients receiving combination chemotherapy with doxorubicin and cyclophosphamide 7 months to 8 years after drug initiation (28). In addition, progressive edema and erythema of the hands followed by induration and skin tightening that later progressed to generalized skin tightening, sclerodactyly of the fingers, and microstomia, has been reported after cycle 2 of topotecan in one patient with ovarian cancer. ANA was 1:640 in a speckled pattern; however, all other autoantibodies were negative including anti-topoisomerase, (Scl70) and there was no internal organ involvement. Topoisomerase binding by topotecan may be involved in this pathogenesis (46). A breast cancer patient receiving the aromatase inhibitor anastrozole developed lichen sclerosus et atrophicus, theorized to be due to lowered estrogen state, and was treated with high-potency topical steroids and low-dose vaginal estrogen (10 mcg estradiol vaginal tablets inserted twice weekly) (29).

Localized sclerosis has also been reported with intravesical instillation of mitomycin C for bladder cancer (30), and with isolated limb perfusion (ILP) therapy with melphalan for soft tissue sarcoma (31). A subcutaneous fat necrosis with sclerosis can occur after transcatheter arterial chemoembolization (TACE) therapy with drug-eluting beads for hepatocellular carcinoma (32).

Targeted Therapy–Related Sclerotic Reactions

Small Molecule Kinase Inhibitors

The tyrosine kinase inhibitor sunitinib has been associated with painful inflammatory edema of the hands and feet, evolving into sclerodermatous skin and joint swelling in one patient. The onset of the eruption was 15 weeks after starting sunitinib 37.5 mg daily. Autoantibodies were negative, and the patient was treated with prednisolone 15 mg daily, topical betamethasone dipropionate twice daily, and oral methotrexate 6 mg/week. The sclerosis recurred with sunitinib rechallenge (33). The BRAF inhibitor vemurafenib has also been associated with sclerotic changes, and 9.4% of patients receiving vemurafenib for metastatic melanoma may develop sclerotic nodules and contractures on the palms consistent with Dupuytren-like palmoplantar fibromatosis. This can occur 4–17 months after initiation of treatment (34). The pathogenesis is unclear, but hypothesized to be due to possible paradoxical activation of the MAP-kinase pathway in BRAF wild-type cells such as fibroblasts, or elevated interferon-gamma, CCL4, and tumor necrosis factor secretion due to BRAF inhibition. In three of the patients, the fibrosis resolved after discontinuation of medication.

Immunotherapy-Related Sclerodermatous Skin Reactions

Programmed Cell Death Protein 1 (PD-1) Inhibitors

Cutaneous immune-related adverse events (irAEs) are common with the use of immunotherapy, and such reactions may include sclerotic skin reactions (35). The PD-1 inhibitor pembrolizumab has been reported to be associated with sclerodermatous skin changes in two patients with BRAF-positive metastatic melanoma. These patients presented after cycle 5 and 13 with initial swelling and stiffness of the extremities followed by indurated skin. The reaction can develop and progress even after discontinuation of immunotherapy. One patient had accompanying Raynaud's and pulmonary symptoms with CT scan showing pneumonitis with ground glass infiltrates. Skin biopsy revealed mild fibrosis and sclerosis with trapping of adnexal structures and minimal lymphocytic inflammation. In these cases, autoantibodies were negative, and no patients had other stigmata of systemic sclerosis such as GI symptoms or capillary nailfold findings. Treatment options include prednisone 1 mg/kg daily intravenous immunoglobulin (0.4 mg/kg for 5 days every month), mycophenolate mofetil 1000 mg twice daily, and hydroxychloroquine (200 mg twice daily).

Patients receiving PD-1 inhibitors may also develop lichen sclerosus or morphea. Nivolumab has been associated with sclerosis of the skin in a patient who previously had 6 years of remission from a prior diagnosis of morphea. The patient developed pruritic shiny atrophic white- and lilac-colored atrophic round plaques two months after initiation of nivolumab for metastatic lung adenocarcinoma (36). A skin biopsy revealed lichen sclerosus with underlying morphea.

Radiation-Induced Sclerosis

Radiation therapy can lead to several types of skin sclerosis, which may be difficult to distinguish from cutaneous metastatic disease or skin infections such as cellulitis.

In the acute period, radiation to the breast can cause a subcutaneous or fascial fibrosis termed radiation-induced fibrosis, which usually develops quickly in the first 3 months after treatment (37).

Delayed sclerotic reactions may also occur. Lichen sclerosus et atrophicus can develop 2–12 years after treatment with ionizing radiation for breast cancer (38,39). The cutaneous changes present as ivory to white atrophic shiny plaques with telangiectasias restricted to the site of prior radiation therapy, and rarely can progress to involve skin outside of the radiated areas.

Vulvar lichen sclerosus et atrophicus has been reported more than one year after treatment with external beam radiation (45 Gy in 25 fractions) followed by a high-dose rate of vaginal cuff brachytherapy (25 Gy in 5 fractions) therapy for a squamous cell carcinoma of the vagina (40). Treatment with high-potency class 1 topical steroids can be helpful.

Radiation-induced localized scleroderma (morphea) occurs in an estimated 1–2 per 1000 (0.2%) patients after radiation therapy for breast cancer, and presents as painful, erythematous indurated plaques within the field of radiation, usually arising months to years after completion of radiation therapy (41,42). The initial inflammatory plaques later become sclerotic, indurated, and hyperpigmented.

The sclerotic reaction does not appear to be related to dose of radiation or acute radiation dermatitis during therapy. The pathogenesis is unclear, but postulated to be due to radiation-induced production of Th2 cytokines that stimulate production of TGF-beta and production of collagen and other extracellular matrix proteins.

Treatment for radiation-induced sclerotic skin reactions include anti-inflammatory agents such as topical, intralesional, or systemic corticosteroids; pentoxifylline; or antioxidant treatment with superoxide disumutase, tocopherol (vitamin E), or PTX-vitamin E combination (43). Other treatments may include

TABLE 6.1

Cancer Therapeutics Associated with Sclerotic Reactions

Drug Class	Drug/Therapy
Alkylating	Carboplatin
Antimetabolite	Capecitabine
	5-Fluorouracil
	Tegafur
	Pemetrexed
	Gemcitabine
	Hydroxyurea
Topoisomerase-interacting	Topotecan
Antimicrotubule	Paclitaxel
	Docetaxel
Small molecule multikinase inhibitors	Sunitinib
	Vemurafenib
Immunotherapy	Interferon
	Nivolumab
	Pembrolizumab
Aromatase inhibitor	Anastrozole
Other	Bleomycin
	Doxorubicin
	Chemoembolization
	Radiation
	Mitomycin C
	Melphalan

UVA-1 therapy (44), topical calcineurin inhibitors, methotrexate, or other immunosuppressive medications including colchicine, penicillamine, and photopheresis (45) (Table 6.1).

REFERENCES

1. Finch WR et al. Bleomycin-induced scleroderma. *J Rheumatol* 1980;7:651–9.
2. Cohen IS et al. Cutaneous toxicity of bleomycin therapy. *Arch Dermatol* 1973;107(4):553–5.
3. Kerr LD, Spiera H. Scleroderma in association with the use of bleomycin: A report of 3 cases. *J Rheumatol* 1992;19:294–6.
4. Yamamoto T. Bleomycin and the skin. *Br J Dermatol* 2006;155(5):869–75.
5. Takeda A et al. Immunohistochemical localization of the neutral cysteine protease bleomycin hydrolase in human skin. *Arch Dermatol Res* 1999;291:238–40.
6. Yamamoto T et al. Animal model of sclerotic skin. I: Local injections of bleomycin induce sclerotic skin mimicking scleroderma. *J Invest Dermatol* 1999;112(4):456–62.
7. Koca SS et al. The protective effects of bevacizumab in bleomycin-induced experimental scleroderma. *Adv Clin Exp Med* 2016;25(2):249–53.
8. Kim KH et al. A case of bleomycin-induced scleroderma. *J Korean Med Sci* 1996;11(5):454–6.
9. Battafarano DF et al. Docetaxel (Taxotere) associated scleroderma-like changes of the lower extremities. A report of three cases. *Cancer* 1995;76:110–5.
10. Kawakami T, Tsutsumi Y, Soma Y. Limited cutaneous systemic sclerosis induced by paclitaxel in a patient with breast cancer. *Arch Dermatol* 2009;145(1):97–8.
11. Itoh M et al. Taxane-induced scleroderma. *Br J Dermatol* 2007;156(2):363–7.
12. Konishi Y et al. Scleroderma-like cutaneous lesions induced by paclitaxel and carboplatin for ovarian carcinoma, not a single course of carboplatin, but re-induced and worsened by previously administrated paclitaxel. *J Obstet Gynaecol Res* 2010;36(3):693–6.

13. Winkelmann RR et al. Paclitaxel-induced diffuse cutaneous sclerosis: A case with associated esophagealdysmotility, Raynaud's phenomenon, and myositis. *Int J Dermatol* 2016;55(1):97–100.
14. Capecitabine package insert. https://www.gene.com/download/pdf/xeloda_prescribing.pdf.
15. Trindade F et al. Hand-foot syndrome with sclerodactyly-like changes in a patient treated with capecitabine. *Am J Dermatopathol* 2008;30(2):172–3.
16. Lee SD et al. Hand-foot syndrome with scleroderma-like change induced by the oral capecitabine: A case report. *Korean J Intern Med* 2007;22:109–12.
17. Saif MW et al. Scleroderma in a patient on capecitabine: Is this a variant of hand-foot syndrome? *Cureus* 2016;8(6):e663.
18. Kono T et al. Scleroderma-like reaction induced by uracil-tegafur (UFT), a second-generation anticancer agent. *J Am Acad Dermatol* 2000;42(3):519–20.
19. Narasimhan P et al. Serious hand-and-foot syndrome in black patients treated with capecitabine: Report of 3 cases and review of the literature. *Cutis* 2004;73(2):101–6.
20. Zhang RX et al. Celecoxib can prevent capecitabine-related hand-foot syndrome in stage II and III colorectal cancer patients: Result of a single-center, prospective randomized phase III trial. *Ann Oncol* 2012;23(5):1348–53.
21. Eguia B et al. Skin toxicities compromise prolonged pemetrexed treatment. *J Thorac Oncol* 2011;6(12):2083–9.
22. Shuster M et al. Lipodermatosclerosis secondary to pemetrexed use. *J Thorac Oncol* 2015;10(3): e11–2.
23. Clarke SJ et al. Phase II trial of pemetrexed disodium (ALIMTA, LY231514) in chemotherapy-naïve patients with advanced non-small-cell lung cancer. *Ann Oncol* 2002;13(5):737–41.
24. Aapro MS, Martin C, Hatty S. Gemcitabine: A safety review. *Anticancer Drugs* 1998;9:191–201.
25. Bessis D et al. Gemcitabine-associated scleroderma-like changes of the lower extremities. *J Am Acad Dermatol* 2004;51(2 Suppl):S73–6.
26. Clowse ME, Wigley FM. Digital necrosis related to carboplatin and gemcitabine therapy in systemic sclerosis. *J Rheumatol* 2003;30(6):1341–3.
27. García-Martínez FJ et al. Scleroderma-like syndrome due to hydroxyurea. *Clin Exp Dermatol* 2012;37(7):755–8.
28. Alexandrescu DT, Bhagwati NS, Wiernik PH. Chemotherapy-induced scleroderma: A pleiomorphic syndrome. *Clin Exp Dermatol* 2005;30(2):141–5.
29. Potter JE, Moore KA. Lichen sclerosus in a breast cancer survivor on an aromatase inhibitor: A case report. *J Gen Intern Med* 2013;28(4):592–5.
30. Calistru AM et al. Pseudoscleroderma possibly induced by intravesical instillation of mitomycin C. *J Am Acad Dermatol* 2010;63(6):e116–8.
31. Landau M et al. Reticulate scleroderma after isolated limb perfusion with melphalan. *J Am Acad Dermatol* 1998;39(6):1011–2.
32. Kim HY et al. Supraumbilical subcutaneous fat necrosis after transcatheter arterial chemoembolization with drug-eluting beads: Case report and review of the literature. *Cardiovasc Intervent Radiol* 2013;36(1):276–9.
33. Ohtsuka T. Sunitinib-induced hand-foot syndrome in a renal cell carcinoma: A sclerodermatous and rheumatoid arthritis-like case. *J Dermatol* 2012;39(11):943–4.
34. Vandersleyen V et al. Vemurafenib-associated Dupuytren- and Ledderhose palmoplantar fibromatosis in metastatic melanoma patients. *J Eur Acad Dermatol Venereol* 2016;30(7):1133–5.
35. Barbosa NS et al. Scleroderma induced by pembrolizumab: A case series. *Mayo Clin Proc* 2017;92(7):1158–63.
36. Alegre-Sánchez A et al. Relapse of morphea during Nivolumab therapy for lung adenocarcinoma. *Actas Dermosifiliogr* 2017;108(1):69–70.
37. Rodemann HP, Bamberg M. Cellular basis of radiation-induced fibrosis. *Radiother Oncol* 1995;35(2):83–90.
38. Vujovic O. Lichen sclerosus in a radiated breast. *CMAJ* 2010;182(18):E860.
39. Yates VM, King CM, Dave VK. Lichen sclerosus et atrophicus following radiation therapy. *Arch Dermatol* 1985;121(8):1044–7.
40. Edwards LR et al. Radiation-induced lichen sclerosus of the vulva: First report in the medical literature. *Wien Med Wochenschr* 2017;167(3–4):74–7.

41. Dyer BA, Hodges MG, Mayadev JS. Radiation-induced morphea: An under-recognized complication of breast irradiation. *Clin Breast Cancer* 2016 Aug;16(4):e141–3.

42. Spalek M, Jonska-Gmyrek J, Gałecki J. Radiation-induced morphea—A literature review. *J Eur Acad Dermatol Venereol* 2015;29(2):197–202.

43. Delanian S, Lefaix JL. Current management for late normal tissue injury: Radiation-induced fibrosis and necrosis. *Semin Radiat Oncol* 2007;17(2):99–107.

44. Kroft EB et al. Ultraviolet A phototherapy for sclerotic skin diseases: A systematic review. *J Am Acad Dermatol* 2008;59(6):1017–30.

45. Fett N, Werth VP. Update on morphea: Part II. Outcome measures and treatment. *J Am Acad Dermatol* 2011;64(2):231–42, quiz 243–4.

46. Ene-Stroescu D, Ellman MH, Peterson CE. Topotecan and the development of scleroderma or a scleroderma-like illness. *Arthritis Rheum* 2002;46(3):844–5.

7

Hand-Foot Reactions

Mathew R. Birnbaum, Loren G. Franco, and Beth N. McLellan

Hand-Foot Syndrome

Epidemiology

Hand-foot syndrome (HFS) was first described in 1974 as a complication following mitotane therapy (1). This eruption, also referred to as palmoplantar erythrodysesthesia, is most commonly caused by cytotoxic chemotherapies, specifically pegylated liposomal doxorubicin (PLD), capecitabine, docetaxel, and 5-fluorouracil (5-FU) (2). The incidence of HFS varies between the use of single agents, with PLD and capecitabine having the highest reported incidence at 40–50% and 50–60%, respectively (Table 7.1) (3). When certain agents are used in combination, such as doxorubicin and continuous 5-FU, the incidence is appreciably higher at 89% (3). The likelihood of developing HFS seems to increase in a dose-dependent fashion as drugs and formulations with longer half-lives and prolonged serum drug levels are associated with higher incidences. This is thought to be one factor contributing to the higher rates of HFS following treatment with PLD (half-life 3–4 days) versus non-liposome-encapsulated doxorubicin (half-life 30 hours). The higher incidence of HFS following continuous infusion of 5-FU compared with a bolus further supports this dose-dependent relationship. Similarly, 5-FU prodrugs, such as capecitabine, have higher rates of HFS, presumably due to their higher sustained tissue drug levels (4).

Other risk factors associated with the development of HFS include drug dosage, genetic variations related to drug metabolism, and female sex (5). Interestingly, studies have suggested developing HFS may portend a prognostic benefit in the setting of breast cancer (6,7). One study investigating breast cancer patients on bevacizumab and capecitabine found that the occurrence of HFS was associated with a reduced risk of death and disease progression by 56% and 44%, respectively (7). More research is needed to adequately support these findings, as variables like median cumulative dose differed between the cohorts.

Pathogenesis

The pathogenesis of HFS is not fully understood and different inciting agents may have distinct causative mechanisms (2). However, studies have shown that direct keratinocyte toxicity may be a shared underlying mechanism. Following infusion, PLD initially concentrates around the superficial and deep portions of the eccrine sweat glands and later permeates to the stratum corneum, most notably on the palms and soles where the concentration of eccrine glands are the highest. PLD in particular seems to favor excretion via the sweat because of its hydrophilic coating. This ultimately leads to an accumulation of PLD in the thick stratum corneum causing the release of toxic free radicals and oxidative damage (8). Animal models show that the oxidative damage may be related to doxorubicin's interaction with copper ions in the skin, leading to the production of reactive oxygen species, the release of inflammatory cytokines, and keratinocyte apoptosis. These studies identified interleukin (IL)-8, IL-1β, IL-1α, and IL-6 as mediating chemokines, which may serve as possible therapeutic targets (9). The higher concentration of eccrine ducts in the palms and soles along with the vascular anatomy, temperature gradient, and high cell turnover of these areas may help explain the observed palmoplantar distribution of HFS, at least in the case of PLD (10).

TABLE 7.1

HFS Incidence

	All Grade	High Grade
Doxorubicin + continuous 5-fluorouracil (3)	89%	24%
Pegylated liposomal doxorubicin (3)	40–50%	1–20%
Doxorubicin (3,4)	22–29%	
Capecitabine (3)	50–60%	11–24%
Docetaxel (3,4)	6–58%	
5-fluorouracil (3,4)		
Continuous infusion	34%	7%
Bolus	6–13%	0.5%
Cytarabine (3,4)	14–33%	

The distribution of HFS may be further explained by keratinocyte enzyme variations at different anatomical areas. Keratinocytes in the palms and soles demonstrate increased thymidine phosphorylase activity, an enzyme responsible for converting the prodrug capecitabine into the active 5-FU (10,11). Mouse models have shown that the metabolites of capecitabine and 5-FU, not the precursor molecules, cause apoptosis through mitochondrial and/or ion channel dysfunction (12). The potential role or 5-FU metabolites and dihydropyrimidine dehydrogenase (DFP) (13) in HFS has been further supported by studies that show higher rates of HFS in patients either with DPD deficiencies or treated with DPD inhibitors (14).

Research has also implicated certain genetic polymorphisms with increased rates and severity of HFS. Cytidine deaminase (CDD) gene is a gene that encodes cytidine deaminase, an enzyme involved in the purine salvage pathway. Cytidine deaminase participates in converting the prodrug capecitabine into 5-FU. Genetic polymorphisms in the promoter region of CDD that presumably lead to more rapid metabolism of capecitabine into 5-FU have been associated with higher rates of HFS (15). Similarly, polymorphisms in genes related to DNA synthesis and folate levels, like methylenetetrahydrofolate reductase (MTHFR), have been associated with the development of HFS (16).

Clinical Presentation

HFS typically presents within 2–21 days of initiating chemotherapy (17). However, reports have shown that eruptions can occur as late as 10 months with certain agents like oral capecitabine or continuous infusion cytarabine (3,4,18). Patients often report dysesthesia that begins as tingling sensations on the palms and soles that progress into burning pain within days. It is believed that damage to the small nerve fibers lead to the observed decrease in pain and temperature sensation, but preservation of light touch and proprioception (19). In conjunction with the neuropathy, palmoplantar erythema and edema can be seen, predominantly on the lateral aspects of the digits and distal fat pads (Figure 7.1) (20). Hyperpigmentation may also be present in patients with darker Fitzpatrick skin types, particularly when following capecitabine use. In high-grade disease, the erythema can progress to desquamation, erosion, and ulceration. Bullae can also develop (Figure 7.2). There is a unique taxane-specific form of HFS known as periarticular thenar erythema with onycholysis (PATEO) (21). It presents with erythema over the thenar and hypothenar eminences, joints, and Achilles tendon (Figure 7.3).

Histopathology

Although the histopathologic findings in HFS are nonspecific, they resemble the constellation of findings seen in cytotoxic reactions (2). The histological findings generally correlate to the clinical severity. The changes observed in the epidermis range from scattered necrotic keratinocytes with basal layer vacuolar degeneration to full-thickness epidermal necrosis. In the dermis, there can be papillary dermal edema and

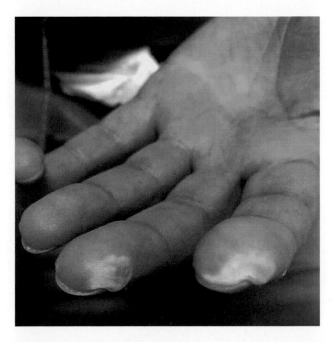

FIGURE 7.1   Palmar erythema and scale in a patient with HFS in a patient on busulfan and cyclophosphamide. (Courtesy of Eugene Balagula, MD.)

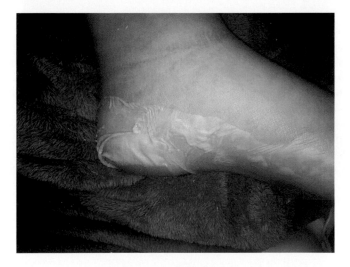

FIGURE 7.2   Hand-foot syndrome with bullae and sloughing in a patient receiving cytarabine, daunorubicin, and etoposide. (Courtesy of Eugene Balagula, MD.)

perivascular infiltrates of lymphocytes and eosinophils. Eccrine squamous syringometaplasia, similar to what is seen in neutrophilic eccrine hidradenitis, has also been reported (3,17,22–24).

Diagnosis

HFS is a clinical diagnosis with the differential diagnosis including contact dermatitis, vasculitis, allergic drug eruptions, erythema multiforme, erythromelalgia, acral bleomycin toxicity, and graft-versus-host disease (GVHD) (5). Infectious etiologies, such as dermatophyte infections, are common in the immunosuppressed and should also be ruled out as they can mimic HFS (2,25).

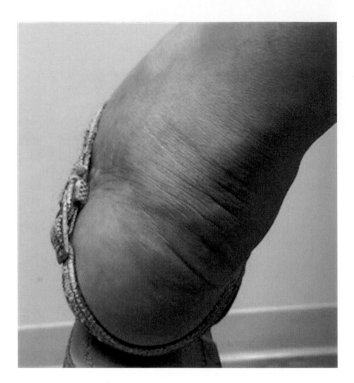

FIGURE 7.3 Violaceous patch over the Achilles tendon in a patient with PATEO.

Classifying and grading the severity of HFS is important and can help dermatologists and oncologists better assess and communicate a patient's clinical status. The World Health Organization (WHO) and National Cancer Institute (NCI) each have a grading system for HFS (Table 7.2) (4,22). Development of grade 3 HFS or higher in both classification schemes may lead to treatment interruption, dose reduction, or discontinuation of the inciting agent. However, even in the more common milder grades of HFS, functional impairment can be significant (5). Validated instruments like the HFS-14 attempt to quantify the effects of HFS on a patient's daily activities (20). Although HFS is not life-threatening and usually resolves within 1–5 weeks of stopping the inciting agent, some long-term sequelae can occur. Repeated episodes of HFS can lead to findings that resemble palmoplantar keratoderma (10). Cases of patients losing their fingerprints have been reported following capecitabine use, but these changes seem to reverse after stopping the medication (26,27). HFS can also increase a patient's risk of developing

TABLE 7.2

NCI Common Terminology Criteria for Adverse Events

Adverse Event	Grade 1	Grade 2	Grade 3	Grade 4	Grade 5
Palmar-plantar erythrodysesthesia syndrome	Minimal skin changes or dermatitis (e.g., erythema, edema, or hyperkeratosis) without pain	Skin changes (e.g., peeling, blisters, bleeding, edema, or hyperkeratosis) with pain; limiting instrumental ADL	Severe skin changes (e.g., peeling blisters, bleeding, edema, or hyperkeratosis) with pain; limiting self-care ADL	—	—

Source: Reproduced from Common Terminology Criteria for Adverse Events (CTCAE), Version 4.0, June 2010, National Institutes of Health, National Cancer Institute. Available at http://evs.nci.nih.gov/ftp1/CTCAE/CTCAE_4.03_2010-06-14_QuickReference_5x7.pdf. Accessed June 2017.

Abbreviations: NCI CTCAE, National Cancer Institute Common Terminology Criteria for Adverse Events; ADL, activities of daily living.

secondary infections. An extreme example is a case report of a death from a pseudomonal superinfection attributed to capecitabine-induced HFS (10).

Treatment and Management

To date the most effective management of HFS is dose modification or treatment interruption with symptoms typically improving in 1–2 weeks (Table 7.3) (10,23,24). When PLD treatments are limited to 10 mg/m^2/week, if HFS does develop, it tends to be mild and easily managed (24,28). If a patient develops grade 2 HFS, it is recommended to delay treatment until symptoms resolve or become grade 1. When grade 3 or 4 HFS occurs, both treatment interruption and dose reduction of 25% or 50%, respectively, is suggested (24). Although there are some large studies, the majority of the treatment literature involves case reports and uncontrolled prospective studies.

Treatment is primarily focused on symptom control with interventions including high-potency topical corticosteroids to reduce inflammation, wound care for erosions and ulceration, topical keratolytics and emollients for hyperkeratosis, and analgesics for pain control. Some reports have found possible benefits with preventive measures, including avoiding both hot water baths and vigorous exercise around the time of drug administration (5). Observed benefits of cooling treatments and vasoconstriction for preventing treatment-related alopecia prompted similar research in HFS. Limiting drug delivery to the extremities via vasoconstriction is thought to mitigate some of the risk of developing HFS. Retrospective and prospective studies have shown lower HFS rates in patients using icepacks or ice water immersion for their palms and soles during PLD infusion (3,10,29). Other studies demonstrated possible benefits with the application of antiperspirant on the palms and soles or the use of frozen gloves and socks during treatment with PLD (30–32). Unfortunately, cooling methods are not feasible when the medication is administered orally or via continuous infusion (2).

A small prospective study showed that after the occurrence grade 2 or higher HFS, oral dexamethasone with future PLD administration led to fewer dose reductions during the subsequent infusions (33). Pyridoxine (vitamin B6) initially was believed to prevent HFS in the setting of PLD, docetaxel, 5-FU, and capecitabine treatment (34). However, more recent studies, including a large meta-analysis, found no benefit to using pyridoxine for any chemotherapy (21,35,36). A randomized controlled trial showed that celecoxib 200 mg twice daily for 14 days during capecitabine therapy reduced the incidence of grade 1 and 2 HFS. It is believed that cyclooxygenase (COX)-mediated vascular damage in the setting of capecitabine explains the potential benefits of celecoxib use for HFS (37). Thus, COX inhibition may be useful in potentially preventing or reducing the severity of HFS.

TABLE 7.3

HFS Management Recommendations

Grade	Symptoms	Findings	Measures: First Occurrence	Measures: Recurrent Episodes
1	None or only slight dysesthesia	Mild redness	Supportive care[a]	Supportive care[a]
2	Dysesthesia but no pain	Severe redness and/or swelling	Delay treatment until grade 1 or less, and consider dose reduction for subsequent courses	Delay treatment until grade 1 or less, and reduce dose 25%
3	Dysesthesia with pain	Severe redness and/or swelling	Delay treatment until grade 1 or less, and reduce dose 25%	Delay treatment until grade 1 or less, and reduce dose an additional 25%
4	Pain and impaired function in the activities of daily living (ADL)	Desquamation, blistering, and ulceration	Delay treatment until grade 1 or less, and reduce dose 50%	Discontinue treatment

Source: From von Moos R et al. *Eur J Cancer* 2008;44(6):781–90. With permission.

[a] Supportive care: Apply emollient cream, wear cotton socks or gloves to bed, avoid skin irritants, extreme temperature, pressure, and friction.

Hand-Foot Skin Reaction

The use of newer targeted anticancer therapies such as multikinase inhibitors (MKIs) has presented its own unique profile of cutaneous adverse events. The clinical findings of these eruptions affecting the palms and soles differ from previously described HFS; this has led to the use of the term HFSR (hand-foot skin reaction), distinguishing it from more classic HFS (38). HFSR has been associated with various mediations including, but not limited to, vemurafenib, regorafenib, cabozantinib, sorafenib, sunitinib, axitinib, and pazopanib (39,40).

Epidemiology

The incidences of all-grade HFSR range from as low as 4.5% with pazopanib treatment to 60% with regorafenib or vemurafenib treatment (Table 7.4) (39,41,42). Combination therapies that target multiple kinases are also associated with a higher incidence of HFSR. When sorafenib, an MKI, is used in conjunction with bevacizumab, an anti-vascular endothelial growth factor (VEGF) antibody, HFSR incidence has been reported to be as high as 79% for all grade and 57% for high-grade reactions (3).

Several risk factors have been identified for the development of HFSR. In patients treated with sorafenib for clear-cell renal cell carcinoma (RCC), development of grade 2 or higher HFSR was correlated with female gender, good performance status, higher pretreatment white blood cell counts, lung and liver metastases, and multiple organ involvement (43).

Several genetic polymorphisms have been associated with increased incidence of HFSR in certain patient populations. One such study demonstrated an increased incidence of HFSR in Korean patients with hepatocellular carcinoma (HCC) treated with sorafenib who have single nucleotide polymorphisms of VEGF or tumor necrosis factor-alpha (TNF-α) (44). Another study in patients treated with sorafenib and/or bevacizumab for various solid tumors observed that both treatment-related hypertension and the presence of a variant allele of VEGFR2, H472Q, independent of each other, portended a higher risk for HFSR (45). Certain malignancies have also been found to be more commonly associated with HFSR, most notably differentiated thyroid cancer (46).

Multiple studies have found an association between survival rates and HFSR in the setting of sorafenib and sunitinib use (47–50).

TABLE 7.4

HFSR Incidence

	Targets	All Grade HFSR	High Grade
Axitinib (64)	VEGFR1/2/3	29.2%	9.6%
Cabozantinib (65,66)	VEGFR2, c-MET, RET, c-KIT, FLT3, Tie-2	35.3%	9.5%
Dabrafenib	RAF (B)	27% (67)	Grade 2 8% (67)
Fruquintinib	Anti-VEGFR	64% (68)	Grade 3 15% (68)
Pazopanib (41)	RAF, VEGFR2/3, PGDFR-β, c-KIT, FLT3, RET	4.5%	1.8%
Regorafenib (42)	VEGFR1/2/3, Tie-2, FGFR-1, PDGFR-α/β, c-KIT, RET, RAF, p38 MAPK	60.5%	20.4%
Sorafenib (69)	VEGFR2/3, PDGFR, RAF (A, B, C), FLT3	59% (70) 33.8	8.9%
Sorafenib + bevacizumab (3)		79%	57%
Sunitinib (71)	VEGFR2, PDGFR, c-KIT, FLT3	18.9%	5.5%
Vemurafenib	RAF (B)	25% (72) 60% (39)	

Source: See further information, see Lacouture ME, McLellan BN, Hand-foot skin reaction induced by multitargeted tyrosine kinase inhibitors, UpToDate.

Abbreviations: c-KIT, mast/stem cell growth factor; FLT3, fms-like tyrosine kinase 3; MAPK, mitogen-activated protein kinase; PDGFR, platelet-derived growth factor receptor; RAF, rapidly accelerated fibrosarcoma; RET, rearranged during transfection; Tie-2, tyrosine-protein kinase receptor; VEGFR, vascular endothelial growth factor receptor.

Pathogenesis

Evidence suggests that VEGF receptor and platelet-derived growth factor (PDGF) inhibition leading to deficient capillary maintenance and repair capabilities may be at least partly responsible (2,51,52). When VEGF and PDGF are inhibited individually, HFSR rarely occurs. However, higher rates of HFSR have been found to occur with combination therapies that simultaneously block both these growth factors (see Table 7.4) (2,3).

Clinical Findings

HFSR typically appears within the first 2–4 weeks of treatment initiation (53). In contrast to HFS, HFSR more commonly involves the soles than the palms. It can also favor sites with increased friction and pressure, such as the interdigital toe web spaces, lateral aspects of the feet, and other areas with friction (Figure 7.4) (2,5). The reaction typically presents as focal, hyperkeratotic callus-like lesions overlying an erythematous base (Figure 7.5). This is in contrast with the more diffuse but well demarcated erythema and scale observed in HFS (2). The lesions can first appear as bullae or blisters and when present, and are often found on the heels, fingertips, and over joints (Figures 7.6 and 7.7) (52). HFSR can also cause paresthesia, pain, decreased heat tolerance, and, in severe cases, may limit a patient's ability to perform activities of daily living like dressing and grooming oneself (53).

Diagnosis

HFSR is a clinical diagnosis and the NCI system is used to grade the severity (Table 7.2) (22,24). It is important to keep in mind the limitations of this tool, as it was not developed specifically for HFSR. Moreover, the grading may be incongruous with a patient's perception of the severity of the eruption (54).

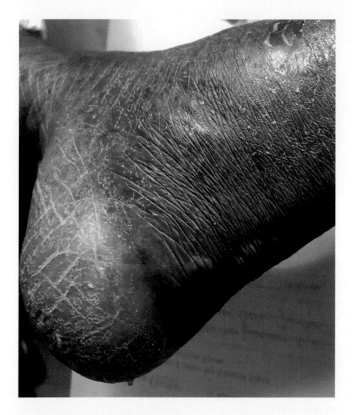

FIGURE 7.4 HFSR over an area of friction from boot in a patient on cabozantinib.

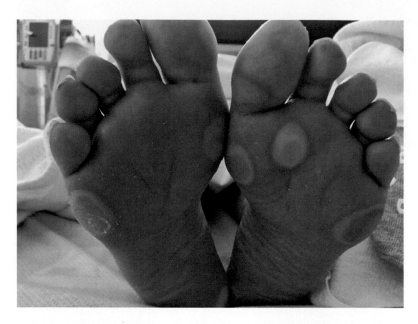

FIGURE 7.5   HFSR in a patient on regorafenib.

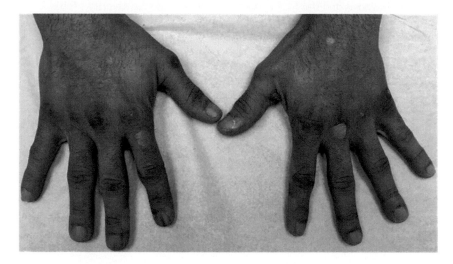

FIGURE 7.6   HFSR in a patient on cabozantinib.

Treatment and Management

The most successful approach to management includes multidisciplinary care involving the patient, oncologist, dermatologist, podiatrist, and nurse. Topical keratolytic agents can be used for all grades of HFSR to treat the observed hyperkeratosis. Urea 10–40%, ammonium lactate 6–12%, or salicylic acid 5–10% can be applied focally to involved lesions, avoiding non-intact skin to minimize possible discomfort (52). Examining the patient to identify sources of friction or ill-fitting clothing or shoes is crucial to minimizing exacerbating factors.

In lower grade HFSR, pain can be treated with topical lidocaine 2–6% in gels, creams, or patches. For grade 2 or higher HFSR, systemic medications, including nonsteroidal anti-inflammatory drugs (NSAIDs), opioids, or *gamma*-Aminobutyric acid (GABA) agonists can be used for pain control (52). Super potent topical steroids are recommended for treatment of the inflamed, erythematous areas of

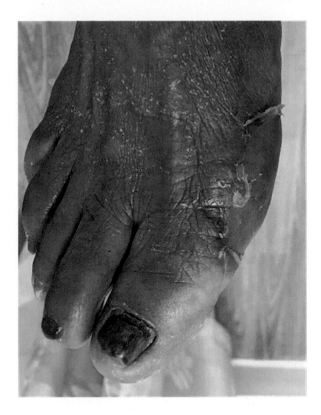

FIGURE 7.7 HFSR in a patient on lenvatinib.

HFSR. Small studies and translational research have found potential benefits with topical sildenafil (55), heparin-containing ointments (56), hydrocolloid dressings containing ceramide (57), and narrowband UVB phototherapy (58), but more research is needed.

A stepwise approach to HFSR is shown in Table 7.5 (59).

Prophylactic measures can help reduce the risk of HFSR. Before initiating treatment with a kinase-targeted therapy, a patient's hands and feet should be examined for existing hyperkeratotic lesions and debrided by a podiatrist or dermatologist. Patients can be counseled on at-home practices like using a pumice stone for gentle exfoliation, keeping hands and feet well-moisturized with bland emollients, and being mindful of potential friction points from their clothing or footwear (52,60). A large randomized control study in patients with advanced hepatocellular carcinoma starting sorafenib assessed the effect of prophylactic 10% urea cream 3 times a day on HSFR incidence. The results showed lower rates of any grade and grade 3 HFSR when comparing the intervention group to the control group (56% vs. 76%, any grade; 20.7% vs. 29.2%, high grade) (61). However, study limitations, such as the control group not receiving any cream, obscures whether the urea or the emollient base was related to changes in HFSR incidence (62). Another recent retrospective study found that prophylactic oral dexamethasone 2 mg delayed dose modifications and decreased the incidence of grade 3 HFSR (3.2% vs. 25.7% in the control) (63).

Conclusion

Continued research in HFS and HFSR will hopefully allow clinicians to better prevent and manage these conditions. As newer anticancer therapies are developed, the incidence and clinical presentation of reactions affecting the palms and soles may continue to evolve. Future research and discoveries in

TABLE 7.5

HFSR Management Algorithm

Severity	Intervention
Grade 0	• Podiatry consultation • Moisturizers • Consider keratolytics (i.e., urea-based cream application three times a day) • Measures to minimize pressure and friction (i.e., thick cotton socks, well-fitting shoes, avoid running)
Grade 1	• Follow above recommendations • Add topical analgesics • Continue anticancer agent at current dose and monitor for change in severity • Reassess after two weeks (either by healthcare professional or patient self-report); if reactions worsen or do not improve, proceed to next step
Grade 2	• Continue above recommendations • Add high-potency topical corticosteroid (i.e., clobetasol propionate 0.05% ointment) • Continue anticancer agent at current dose and monitor for change in severity • Reassess after 2 weeks (either by healthcare professional or patient self-report); if reactions worsen or do not improve, proceed to next step
Grade 3 or intolerable grade 2	• Continue topical medications as above • Hold TKI for 7 days or until HFSR symptoms resolve then resume at a lower dose as per prescribing information • If reaction worsens or does not improve, dose interruption or discontinuation per prescribing information may be necessary

Source: For further information, see Lacouture ME, McLellan BN, Hand-foot skin reaction induced by multitargeted tyrosine kinase inhibitors, UpToDate.

Abbreviations: TKI, tyrosine kinase inhibitor; HFSR, hand-foot skin reaction.

genomics and polymorphisms will likely change and improve our understanding of both HFS and HFSR. It remains to be determined how clinicians will use the likely prognostic significance of HFS and HFSR in their management and treatment of afflicted patients.

REFERENCES

1. Zuehlke RL. Erythematous eruption of the palms and soles associated with mitotane therapy. *Dermatologica* 1974;148(2):90–2.
2. Miller KK, Gorcey L, McLellan BN. Chemotherapy-induced hand-foot syndrome and nail changes: A review of clinical presentation, etiology, pathogenesis, and management. *J Am Acad Dermatol* 2014;71(4):787–94.
3. Degen A et al. The hand-foot-syndrome associated with medical tumor therapy—Classification and management. *J Dtsch Dermatol Ges* 2010;8(9):652–61.
4. Nagore E, Insa A, Sanmartin O. Antineoplastic therapy-induced palmar plantar erythrodysesthesia ("hand-foot") syndrome. Incidence, recognition and management. *Am J Clin Dermatol* 2000;1(4):225–34.
5. Lipworth AD, Robert C, Zhu AX. Hand-foot syndrome (hand-foot skin reaction, palmar-plantar erythrodysesthesia): Focus on sorafenib and sunitinib. *Oncology* 2009;77(5):257–71.
6. Azuma Y et al. Significant association between hand-foot syndrome and efficacy of capecitabine in patients with metastatic breast cancer. *Biol Pharm Bull* 2012;35(5):717–24.
7. Zielinski C et al. Predictive role of hand-foot syndrome in patients receiving first-line capecitabine plus bevacizumab for HER2-negative metastatic breast cancer. *Br J Cancer* 2016;114(2):163–70.
8. Martschick A et al. The pathogenetic mechanism of anthracycline-induced palmar-plantar erythrodysesthesia. *Anticancer Res* 2009;29(6):2307–13.
9. Yokomichi N et al. Pathogenesis of hand-foot syndrome induced by PEG-modified liposomal doxorubicin. *Hum Cell* 2013;26(1):8–18.

10. Hoesly FJ, Baker SG, Gunawardane ND, Cotliar JA. Capecitabine-induced hand-foot syndrome complicated by pseudomonal superinfection resulting in bacterial sepsis and death: Case report and review of the literature. *Arch Dermatol* 2011;147(12):1418–23.

11. Milano G et al. Candidate mechanisms for capecitabine-related hand-foot syndrome. *Br J Clin Pharmacol* 2008;66(1):88–95.

12. Chen M et al. The contribution of keratinocytes in capecitabine-stimulated hand-foot-syndrome. *Environ Toxicol Pharmacol* 2017;49:81–8.

13. Kwakman JJM et al. Tolerability of the oral fluoropyrimidine S-1 after hand-foot syndrome-related discontinuation of capecitabine in western cancer patients. *Acta Oncol* 2017;56(7):1023–6.

14. Yen-Revollo JL, Goldberg RM, McLeod HL. Can inhibiting dihydropyrimidine dehydrogenase limit hand-foot syndrome caused by fluoropyrimidines? *Clin Cancer Res* 2008;14(1):8–13.

15. Caronia D et al. A polymorphism in the cytidine deaminase promoter predicts severe capecitabine-induced hand-foot syndrome. *Clin Cancer Res* 2011;17(7):2006–13.

16. Roberto M et al. Evaluation of 5-fluorouracil degradation rate and Pharmacogenetic profiling to predict toxicity following adjuvant Capecitabine. *Eur J Clin Pharmacol* 2017;73(2):157–64.

17. Bolognia JL, Cooper DL, Glusac EJ. Toxic erythema of chemotherapy: A useful clinical term. *J Am Acad Dermatol* 2008;59(3):524–9.

18. Baack BR, Burgdorf WH. Chemotherapy-induced acral erythema. *J Am Acad Dermatol* 1991;24(3):457–61.

19. Stubblefield MD, Custodio CM, Kaufmann P, Dickler MN. Small-fiber neuropathy associated with capecitabine (Xeloda)-induced hand-foot syndrome: A case report. *J Clin Neuromuscul Dis* 2006;7(3):128–32.

20. Sibaud V et al. HFS-14, a specific quality of life scale developed for patients suffering from hand-foot syndrome. *Oncologist* 2011;16(10):1469–78.

21. von Gruenigen V et al. A double-blind, randomized trial of pyridoxine versus placebo for the prevention of pegylated liposomal doxorubicin-related hand-foot syndrome in gynecologic oncology patients. *Cancer* 2010;116(20):4735–43.

22. Common Terminology Criteria for Adverse Events (CTCAE), Version 4.0, June 2010, National Institutes of Health, National Cancer Institute [cited 2017 June 23]. Available from: http://evs.nci.nih.gov/ftp1/CTCAE/CTCAE_4.03_2010-06-14_QuickReference_5x7.pdf.

23. Farr KP, Safwat A. Palmar-plantar erythrodysesthesia associated with chemotherapy and its treatment. *Case Rep Oncol* 2011;4(1):229–35.

24. von Moos R et al. Pegylated liposomal doxorubicin-associated hand-foot syndrome: Recommendations of an international panel of experts. *Eur J Cancer* 2008;44(6):781–90.

25. Wang JZ, Cowley A, McLellan BN. Differentiating hand-foot syndrome from tinea in patients receiving chemotherapy. *Acta Oncol* 2016;55(8):1061–4.

26. van Doorn L, Veelenturf S, Binkhorst L, Bins S, Mathijssen R. Capecitabine and the risk of fingerprint loss. *JAMA Oncology* 2017;3(1):122–3.

27. Wong M, Choo SP, Tan EH. Travel warning with capecitabine. *Ann Oncol* 2009;20(7):1281.

28. Gressett SM, Stanford BL, Hardwicke F. Management of hand-foot syndrome induced by capecitabine. *J Oncol Pharm Pract* 2006;12(3):131–41.

29. Mangili G, Petrone M, Gentile C, De Marzi P, Vigano R, Rabaiotti E. Prevention strategies in palmar-plantar erythrodysesthesia onset: The role of regional cooling. *Gynecol Oncol* 2008;108(2):332–5.

30. Templeton AJ et al. Prevention of palmar-plantar erythrodysesthesia with an antiperspirant in breast cancer patients treated with pegylated liposomal doxorubicin (SAKK 92/08). *Breast* 2014;23(3):244–9.

31. Scotte F et al. Multicenter study of a frozen glove to prevent docetaxel-induced onycholysis and cutaneous toxicity of the hand. *Am J Clin Oncol* 2005;23(19):4424–9.

32. Scotte F et al. Matched case-control phase 2 study to evaluate the use of a frozen sock to prevent docetaxel-induced onycholysis and cutaneous toxicity of the foot. *Cancer* 2008;112(7):1625–31.

33. Drake RD, Lin WM, King M, Farrar D, Miller DS, Coleman RL. Oral dexamethasone attenuates Doxil-induced palmar-plantar erythrodysesthesias in patients with recurrent gynecologic malignancies. *Gynecol Oncol* 2004;94(2):320–4.

34. Corrie PG et al. A randomised study evaluating the use of pyridoxine to avoid capecitabine dose modifications. *Br J Cancer* 2012;107(4):585–7.

35. Jo SJ, Shin H, Jo S, Kwon O, Myung SK. Prophylactic and therapeutic efficacy of pyridoxine supplements in the management of hand–foot syndrome during chemotherapy: A meta-analysis. *Clin Exp Dermatol* 2015;40(3):260–70.

36. Yap Y et al. Predictors of hand-foot syndrome and pyridoxine for prevention of capecitabine–induced hand-foot syndrome: A randomized clinical trial. *JAMA Oncology* 2017;3(11):1538–45.

37. Zhang RX et al. Celecoxib can prevent capecitabine-related hand-foot syndrome in stage II and III colorectal cancer patients: Result of a single-center, prospective randomized phase III trial. *Ann Oncol* 2012;23(5):1348–53.

38. Porta C, Paglino C, Imarisio I, Bonomi L. Uncovering Pandora's vase: The growing problem of new toxicities from novel anticancer agents. The case of sorafenib and sunitinib. *Clin Exp Med* 2007;7(4):127–34.

39. Boussemart L et al. Prospective study of cutaneous side-effects associated with the BRAF inhibitor vemurafenib: A study of 42 patients. *Ann Oncol* 2013;24(6):1691–7.

40. Massey PR, Okman JS, Wilkerson J, Cowen EW. Tyrosine kinase inhibitors directed against the vascular endothelial growth factor receptor (VEGFR) have distinct cutaneous toxicity profiles: A meta-analysis and review of the literature. *Support Care Cancer* 2015;23(6):1827–35.

41. Balagula Y, Wu S, Su X, Feldman DR, Lacouture ME. The risk of hand foot skin reaction to pazopanib, a novel multikinase inhibitor: A systematic review of literature and meta-analysis. *Investig New Drugs* 2012;30(4):1773–81.

42. Belum V, Wu S, Lacouture ME. Risk of hand-foot skin reaction with the novel multikinase inhibitor regorafenib: A meta-analysis. *Investig New Drugs* 2013;31(4):1078–86.

43. Dranitsaris G, Vincent MD, Yu J, Huang L, Fang F, Lacouture ME. Development and validation of a prediction index for hand-foot skin reaction in cancer patients receiving sorafenib. *Ann Oncol* 2012;23(8):2103–8.

44. Lee JH et al. Genetic predisposition of hand-foot skin reaction after sorafenib therapy in patients with hepatocellular carcinoma. *Cancer* 2013;119(1):136–42.

45. Jain L et al. Hypertension and hand-foot skin reactions related to VEGFR2 genotype and improved clinical outcome following bevacizumab and sorafenib. *J Exp Clin Cancer Res* 2010;29:95.

46. Jean GW, Mani RM, Jaffry A, Khan SA. Toxic effects of sorafenib in patients with differentiated thyroid carcinoma compared with other cancers. *JAMA Oncology* 2016;2(4):529–34.

47. Nagyivanyi K et al. Synergistic survival: A new phenomenon connected to adverse events of first-line sunitinib treatment in advanced renal cell carcinoma. *Clin Genitourin Cancer* 2015;14(4):314–22.

48. Nakano K et al. Hand-foot skin reaction is associated with the clinical outcome in patients with metastatic renal cell carcinoma treated with sorafenib. *Jpn J Clin Oncol* 2013;43(10):1023–9.

49. Poprach A et al. Skin toxicity and efficacy of sunitinib and sorafenib in metastatic renal cell carcinoma: A national registry-based study. *Ann Oncol* 2012;23(12):3137–43.

50. Lamarca A, Abdel-Rahman O, Salu I, McNamara MG, Valle JW, Hubner RA. Identification of clinical biomarkers for patients with advanced hepatocellular carcinoma receiving sorafenib. *Clin Transl Oncol* 2017;19(3):364–72.

51. Azad NS et al. Hand-foot skin reaction increases with cumulative sorafenib dose and with combination anti-vascular endothelial growth factor therapy. *Clin Cancer Res* 2009;15(4):1411–6.

52. McLellan B, Ciardiello F, Lacouture ME, Segaert S, Van Cutsem E. Regorafenib-associated hand-foot skin reaction: Practical advice on diagnosis, prevention, and management. *Ann Oncol* 2015;26(10):2017–26.

53. McLellan B, Kerr H. Cutaneous toxicities of the multikinase inhibitors sorafenib and sunitinib. *Dermatol Ther* 2011;24(4):396–400.

54. Trotti A, Colevas AD, Setser A, Basch E. Patient-reported outcomes and the evolution of adverse event reporting in oncology. *J Clin Oncol* 2007;25(32):5121–7.

55. Meadows KL et al. Treatment of palmar-plantar erythrodysesthesia (PPE) with topical sildenafil: A pilot study. *Support Care Cancer* 2015;23(5):1311–9.

56. Li JR et al. Efficacy of a protocol including heparin ointment for treatment of multikinase inhibitor-induced hand-foot skin reactions. *Support Care Cancer* 2013;21(3):907–11.

57. Shinohara N et al. A randomized multicenter phase II trial on the efficacy of a hydrocolloid dressing containing ceramide with a low-friction external surface for hand-foot skin reaction caused by sorafenib in patients with renal cell carcinoma. *Ann Oncol* 2014;25(2):472–6.

58. Hung CT, Chiang CP, Wu BY. Sorafenib-induced psoriasis and hand-foot skin reaction responded dramatically to systemic narrowband ultraviolet B phototherapy. *J Dermatol* 2012;39(12):1076–7.

59. Lacouture ME, McLellan BN. *Hand-foot skin reaction induced by multitargeted tyrosine kinase inhibitors.* UpToDate.
60. Manchen E, Robert C, Porta C. Management of tyrosine kinase inhibitor-induced hand-foot skin reaction: Viewpoints from the medical oncologist, dermatologist, and oncology nurse. *J Support Oncol* 2011;9(1):13–23.
61. Ren Z et al. Randomized controlled trial of the prophylactic effect of urea-based cream on sorafenib-associated hand-foot skin reactions in patients with advanced hepatocellular carcinoma. *J Clin Oncol* 2015;33(8):894–900.
62. Negri FV, Porta C. Urea-based cream to prevent sorafenib-induced hand-and-foot skin reaction: Which evidence? *J Clin Oncol* 2015;33(28):3219–20.
63. Fukuoka S et al. Prophylactic use of oral dexamethasone to alleviate fatigue during regorafenib treatment for patients with metastatic colorectal cancer. *Clin Colorectal Cancer* 2017;16(2):e39–44.
64. Fischer A, Wu S, Ho AL, Lacouture ME. The risk of hand-foot skin reaction to axitinib, a novel VEGF inhibitor: A systematic review of literature and meta-analysis. *Investig New Drugs* 2013;31(3):787–97.
65. Belum VR, Serna-Tamayo C, Wu S, Lacouture ME. Incidence and risk of hand-foot skin reaction with cabozantinib, a novel multikinase inhibitor: A meta-analysis. *Clin Exp Dermatol* 2015;41(1):8–15.
66. Zuo RC et al. Cutaneous adverse effects associated with the tyrosine-kinase inhibitor cabozantinib. *JAMA Dermatology* 2015;151(2):170–7.
67. Long GV et al. Dabrafenib and trametinib versus dabrafenib and placebo for Val600 BRAF-mutant melanoma: A multicentre, double-blind, phase 3 randomised controlled trial. *Lancet* 2015;386(9992):444–51.
68. Xu RH et al. Safety and efficacy of fruquintinib in patients with previously treated metastatic colorectal cancer: A phase Ib study and a randomized double-blind phase II study. *J Hematol Oncol* 2017;10(1):22.
69. Chu D, Lacouture ME, Fillos T, Wu S. Risk of hand-foot skin reaction with sorafenib: A systematic review and meta-analysis. *Acta Oncol* 2008;47(2):176–86.
70. Akaza H et al. A large-scale prospective registration study of the safety and efficacy of sorafenib tosylate in unresectable or metastatic renal cell carcinoma in Japan: Results of over 3200 consecutive cases in post-marketing all-patient surveillance. *Jpn J Clin Oncol* 2015;45(10):953–62.
71. Chu D, Lacouture ME, Weiner E, Wu S. Risk of hand-foot skin reaction with the multitargeted kinase inhibitor sunitinib in patients with renal cell and non-renal cell carcinoma: A meta-analysis. *Clin Genitourin Cancer* 2009;7(1):11–9.
72. Robert C et al. Improved overall survival in melanoma with combined dabrafenib and trametinib. *N Engl J Med* 2015;372(1):30–9.

8

Oral Mucosal Reactions to Anticancer Therapies

Emmanuelle Vigarios and Vincent Sibaud

Introduction

Among the wide range of toxicities induced by anticancer treatments, oral mucositis remains a major and frequent debilitating adverse event associated with cytotoxic chemotherapy and with head and neck radiation therapy (1). Oral mucositis frequently represents a significant burden for patients, negatively impacting their quality of life (2,3). Other chemo- or radio-induced oral adverse events are also well identified, such as dry mouth, taste disturbances, and pigmentary changes.

In contrast, oral adverse events induced by new anticancer treatments (i.e., targeted therapies and immune checkpoint inhibitors) remain poorly characterized (except mTOR inhibitor–associated stomatitis) and have been mainly reported using nonspecific terminology ("stomatitis," "mucosal inflammation," "mucositis"). Yet, oral toxicities induced by targeted therapies often display very characteristic features that clearly differ from the classic oral injuries observed with cytotoxic chemotherapy and/or radiation therapy (Table 8.1). In addition, they frequently affect more than 20% of treated patients and can lead to significant morbidity or permanent treatment discontinuation (4). In the same way, anti-PD-1/PD-L1 immune checkpoint antibodies can be also associated with characteristic oral changes (5–7).

Cytotoxic Chemotherapy

Mucositis

Chemo-induced oral mucositis remains a common, dose-limiting, symptomatically devastating toxicity of chemotherapy (8–20). Approximately 20–40% of patients undergoing chemotherapeutic treatment for solid cancers and about 80% of patients receiving very high doses of chemotherapy before hematopoietic stem cell transplantation (HSCT) will experience some type of mucositis during their first course of treatment. The incidence may increase to more than two-thirds in subsequent cycles, especially when chemotherapy is used in combination. Although mucositis may occur after administration of any form of cytotoxic chemotherapeutic agent, the antimetabolites and alkylating agents have been associated with the highest incidences and degrees of severity of oral mucositis. Examples of the most frequently offending drugs are methotrexate, bleomycin, docetaxel, doxorubicin, fluorouracil, dactinomycin, vinorelbine, cisplatin, carboplatin, irinotecan, cyclophosphamide, etoposide, and paclitaxel. Overall, patients at greatest risk include those treated for hematologic malignancies, patients under 20 years old, patients with preexisting oral disease, and those with a poor nutritional status.

Although epithelial cells are extremely susceptible to drugs that inhibit mitosis or interfere with DNA synthesis, oral mucositis is not the unique consequence of the clonogenic cell death of these rapidly dividing basal cells. Indeed, as initially described by Sonis in a five-step model (10), it has been demonstrated that chemotherapy activates more complex interactions within submucosa cells inducing the generation of damaging reactive oxygen species, the activation of specific transcription factors (e.g., nuclear factor kappa B) and inflammatory signaling pathways (e.g., PI3 K/AKT, SAPK/JNK, toll-like receptors), and the upregulation of proinflammatory cytokines (e.g., TNF-alpha, Il-1 beta, Il-6) (1,10).

TABLE 8.1

Main Oral Changes Induced by Targeted Anticancer Therapies[e]

Class of Targeted Therapies	Drugs	Mechanism of Action/Targets	Clinical Presentation	Mucositis/Stomatitis Approx. Incidences		Other Oral Changes	International Nonproprietary Name
				All Grades %	Grades ≥3%		
mTOR inhibitors	Everolimus + exemestane	STKI[a] targeting mTOR	mIAS: mTOR inhibitor–associated stomatitis (aphthous-like lesions) Nonkeratinized mucosa	62–67	8–13	Dysgeusia Xerostomia	—
	Everolimus			24–64	1–9		Afinitor®
	Temsirolimus			22–26	2–7		Torisel®
EGFR (or HER1) inhibitors	Erlotinib	TKI[b] targeting EGFR	Limited mucositis[c] and aphthous-like lesions	8–20	≤1	Dysgeusia	Tarceva®
	Gefitinib			19–24	≤1		Iressa®
	Cetuximab	Monoclonal antibody targeting EGFR	Nonkeratinized mucosa	7 56–72 (with head and neck radiotherapy)	≤1		Erbitux®
	Panitumumab			5	≤1		Vectibix®
HER inhibitors	Afatinib	TKI targeting EGF (ErbB1), HER2 (ErbB2), ErbB3, and ErbB4 receptors	Limited mucositis and aphthous-like lesions[c]	29–64	3–7	Dysgeusia Xerostomia	Giotrif®
	Dacomitinib	Irreversible TKI targeting EGFR, HER2, and HER4 tyrosine kinases	Nonkeratinized mucosa	37–41	3–4		Under development
	Lapatinib	TKI targeting EGF (ErbB1) and HER2 (ErbB2) receptors		6	1		Tyverb®
	Trastuzumab Emtansine	Monoclonal antibody targeting HER2; antibody-drug conjugate with chemotherapy (emtansine)				Mucosal bleeding and telangiectasia	Kadcyla®
Angiogenesis inhibitors	Sunitinib	TKI targeting VEGFR 1-3, PDGFR α, β, c-KIT, RET, FLT3, CSF-1R	Nonspecific stomatitis Oral dysesthesia	22–27	1–4	Benign migratory glossitis osteonecrosis of jaw	Sutent®
	Cabozantinib	TKI targeting VEGFR, AXL, MET	Aphthous-like lesions	22–29	2	Dysgeusia Xerostomia	Cometriq®
	Sorafenib	TKI targeting VEGFR 2-3, PDGFR β, c-KIT, RET, RAF, FLT3		7–19	0.5–2	Dyschromia (sunitinib)	Nexavar®
	Pazopanib	TKI targeting VEGFR 1-3, PDGFR α-β, c-KIT		14	1		Votrient®
	Axitinib	TKI targeting VEGFR 1-3		15	1		Inlyta®
	Bevacizumab	Monoclonal antibody targeting VEGF				Benign migratory glossitis Osteonecrosis of jaw Mucosal bleeding Delayed wound healing	Avastin®

(Continued)

TABLE 8.1 (*Continued*)

Main Oral Changes Induced by Targeted Anticancer Therapies

Class of Targeted Therapies	Drugs	Mechanism of Action/Targets	Main Oral Toxicities	International Nonproprietary Name
BCR-ABL inhibitors	Imatinib	TKI targeting BCR-ABL (Philadelphia chromosome), PDGFR α β, c-Kit, CSF-1R, SCF receptors	Lichenoid reactions "Blue-gray" hyperpigmentation (hard palate) Dysgeusia	Glivec®
BRAF inhibitors	Dabrafenib Vemurafenib Encorafenib (LGX)	STKI targeting BRAF	Mucosal hyperkeratotic lesions[d] (linea alba, hard palate, gingiva) Gingival hyperplasia Secondary oral squamous cell carcinoma	Tafinlar® Zelboraf® —
ALK inhibitors	Crizotinib	TKI targeting ALK, MET, ROS1	Dysgeusia	Xalkori®
Hedgehog pathway inhibitors	Vismodegib	Targeting SMO protein	Dysgeusia Ageusia	Erivedge®

[a] Serine threonine kinase inhibitor (STKI).

[b] Tyrosine kinase inhibitor (TKI).

[c] Grade ≥3 mucositis is frequent when cetuximab is associated with head and neck radiotherapy for locally advanced squamous cell carcinoma.

[d] These induced lesions do not develop when BRAF inhibitors are associated with MEK inhibitors.

[e] From selected phase I to III trials (drug in monotherapy). Data from Vigarios E, et al. *Support Care Cancer* 2017;25:1713–39.

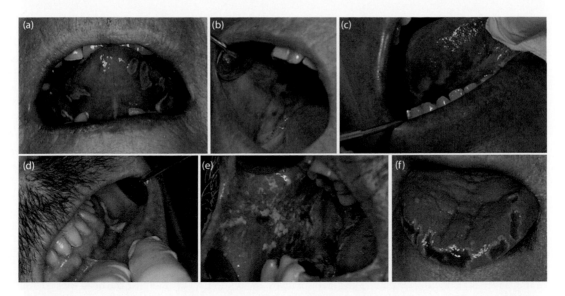

FIGURE 8.1 Chemo-induced mucositis. (a) Mucositis involving the ventral aspect of the tongue (eribulin monotherapy). (b) Poorly circumscribed ulceration with a pseudomembrane on the buccal mucosa (docetaxel, cisplatin, and 5-fluorouracil in combination). (c) Mucositis involving the lateral aspects of the tongue (cisplatin monotherapy). (d) Grade 2 chemo-induced mucositis (busulfan and cyclophosphamide in combination). (e) Pseudomembranous oral candidiasis superinfection in a patient receiving high doses of chemotherapy before HSCT. (f) Herpetic reactivation in a patient receiving capecitabine monotherapy.

Chemotherapy-related mucositis usually starts 4–7 days after the first cycle. It typically involves the nonkeratinized mucosa (floor of the mouth, soft palate, oral mucosa, ventral part of the tongue, lips), with a relative sparing of keratinized areas. The premonitory phase includes erythema and burning. Lesions may evolve to form erosions and ulcerations (1,10,11,13), covered by a pseudomembrane consisting of fibrin, altered leucocytes, and epithelial debris (Figure 8.1a through d). Ulcerations are initially distinct, but may ultimately become diffuse, poorly circumscribed, and confluent. Pain and xerostomia are readily reported by patients. Inference with food/fluid intake is also common. Concomitant gastrointestinal involvement is also frequently noted (1,12,13).

A variety of assessment scales can be employed to grade the severity of the oral mucositis. The most commonly used are the National Cancer Institute (NCI) Common Toxicity Criteria (CTC, version 4.0) and the World Health Organization scale (18) (Table 8.2).

Fungal infections (oral candidiasis; Figure 8.1e) and viral reactivations (herpetic infection; Figure 8.1f) can also be seen in this context (1,13). Finally, mucosal injury may lead to impaired health-related quality

TABLE 8.2

Oral Mucositis Grading Scales

	WHO Scale	National Cancer Institute Common Terminology Criteria for Adverse Events (Version 4.03)
Grade 0	No oral mucositis	—
Grade 1	Erythema and soreness	Asymptomatic or mild symptoms; intervention not indicated
Grade 2	Ulcers; able to eat solids	Moderate pain not interfering with oral intake; modified diet indicated
Grade 3	Ulcers; requires liquid diet (due to mucositis)	Severe pain interfering with oral intake
Grade 4	Ulcers; alimentation not possible (due to mucositis)	Life-threatening consequences; urgent intervention indicated
Grade 5	—	Death

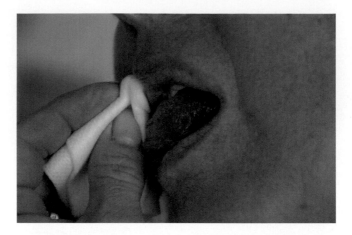

FIGURE 8.2   Oral neutropenic ulcer.

of life, adversely affecting the patient and their relatives. In addition, it may increase the need for systemic analgesics and the length of stay in institutions.

Finally, mucositis induced by chemotherapy should be distinguished from neutropenic ulcers secondary to myelosuppression (Figure 8.2). Clinically, these ulcerated lesions with sharper borders are surrounded by erythema. They can vary in shape, number, and size (14). They also affect keratinized and nonkeratinized mucosae indiscriminately.

Management

Several health professional organizations have reported strategies for management of oral mucositis. Supportive care is mostly palliative (15). The authors of the final version of the European Society for Medical Oncology (ESMO) guidelines have reformatted the content of the Multinational Association of Supportive Care in Cancer and International Society of Oral Oncology (MASCC/ISOO) guidelines in order to further facilitate their use by clinicians (16). Two key strategies for mitigation of oral mucosal injury before and during treatment rely on maintaining optimal nutritional support throughout the entire period of cancer therapy and developing a daily oral hygiene routine (17) (Table 8.3).

No standardized management strategy exists but general symptomatic support and some therapeutic interventions for prevention or treatment can be recommended (based on higher level evidence) or suggested (based on lower level evidence) (1,16,17) (Tables 8.4 through 8.7). However, the ideal management of oral mucositis remains a challenging problem.

Prevention

Early management consists of the promotion of good oral hygiene. First, pretherapeutic oral screening is recommended in order to identify dental or periodontal disease outbreaks and ensure proper treatment. Oral examination is also necessary to eliminate potential sources of trauma (ill-fitting dentures, defective restorations, broken teeth, dental calculus, etc.) and detect preexisting mucosal disease (19). Good oral health also relies on basic oral care interventions (16,17,19) (Table 8.3).

Several agents have been proposed for the prevention of chemo-induced oral mucositis, but their reported efficacy is inconsistent. Oral cryotherapy, zinc supplements, exposure to soft low-level laser therapy (photobiomodulation), or systemic administration of keratinocyte growth factor/palifermin (12,15–17,19) remain only recommended or suggested for the specific indications reported in Tables 8.4 and 8.5. Other coating, antimicrobial, or anti-inflammatory agents described in anecdotal reports and based on low-level studies should not be considered (1,19).

Mucositis Treatment

Pain is the most prominent symptom of oral mucositis and providing relief is fundamental for continuing treatment (12,13,15–17,19,20). In general, no intervention is required for grade 1 mucositis, except for

TABLE 8.3

Basic Oral Care, Oral Hygiene, and Dietary Recommendations

General measures for patients
- Inspect your oral mucosa daily
- Drink ample amounts of fluids
- Before oncologic treatment, have preoperative dental and periodontal screening with treatment as appropriate (elimination of traumatic factors [dental or prosthetic origin], treatment of dental infections)
- During and after treatment, have regular dental and periodontal examinations

Dental and gum care
- Tooth brushing 2 or 3 times a day with an ultrasoft or soft toothbrush with mild fluoride-containing, nonfoaming toothpaste (in case of burning, use minimally flavored toothpaste, for example, children's toothpaste/gel)
- Remove dentures before performing oral care
- Flossing/interdental cleaning after each meal
- Mouth washing with bland solutions 4 to 6 times a day (sterile water, normal saline, or sodium bicarbonate); during the first half-hour after rinsing, avoid eating and drinking
- Cleaning removable dental prostheses; if possible soak the denture for 10 minutes in antimicrobial solution (chlorhexidine 0.2% if available)
- Consider oral moisturizers; be aware that Vaseline/white paraffin should not be used chronically on the lips as this promotes mucosal cell dehydration and occlusion, leading to risk of secondary infection

Avoid
- Alcohol-containing rinses and toothpaste with sodium lauryl sulfate
- Alcohol or peroxidase containing mouthwash products
- Antifungal or antimicrobial products without specific indications

Dietary recommendations
- Frequent drinks between meals
- Chewing slowly
- Diversifying and favoring foods for which flavor is not too distorted
- Further enhancing the flavor of food using seasonings and flavorings, consuming cold foods, and avoiding overly fragrant foods
- Avoid spicy, acidic, hard, crunchy, and/or high temperature food; alcoholic drinks; and tobacco

Source: Vigarios E et al. *Support Care Cancer* 2017;25:1713–39; Lalla RV et al. *Cancer* 2014;120:1453–61.

using mouthwash with bland solutions (sterile water, normal saline, or sodium bicarbonate) and for maintaining a good standard of oral hygiene. Good oral hygiene represents a key factor for alleviating the symptoms of oral mucositis, and basic oral care protocols should be considered as a first-line treatment for reducing the pain and severity of oral mucositis across all cancer modalities. Avoiding hot and spicy food, alcohol, and smoking is also crucial for reducing the severity of oral mucositis (Table 8.3).

For grade 2/3 mucositis, additional mouth rinses should be considered (e.g., 0.2% morphine mouthwash). Systemic analgesics or transdermal fentanyl should be also used to control the pain (1,17). In our experience, a topical steroid mouth rinse (e.g., dexamethasone mouth rinse [0.1 mg/mL]) should be considered as a first-line treatment for diffuse painful mucositis after ruling out an active infection. For limited lesions that can be reached for topical application, high-potency corticosteroids (e.g., clobetasol 0.05% gel or cream) are an alternative (4). In our experience, the association of low-level laser therapy (wavelength of 633–685 or 780–830 nm; power output of between 10 and 150 mW; energy density 2–3 J/cm^2, and no more than 6 J/cm^2 on the tissue surface treated) (20) with topical corticosteroids provides some pain relief after two sessions (48 hours apart) and may promote healing of mucositis. However, these data need to be confirmed by prospective studies.

High-grade mucositis may also require dose adjustments, which leads to resolution of symptoms within 2 weeks of chemotherapy being withdrawn. The severity and/or the recurrence of the lesions, and the time needed for recovering, will determine whether full dosing can be resumed or whether dose reduction or discontinuation is required.

Finally, severe mucositis can severely compromise oral intake. Support from a dietitian, including advice related to dietary supplements, should be considered. Gastrostomy or nasogastric tube feeding can sometimes be required in case of severe lesions (1).

TABLE 8.4

Recommendations for Prevention of Oral Mucositis

Recommendation in Favor of an Intervention	Level of Evidence	Therapy	Cancer
30 minutes of oral cryotherapy	II	Patients receiving bolus-5-fluorouracil chemotherapy	Cancer of any kind
Photobiomodulation (low-level laser therapy; wavelength at 650 nm, power of 40 mW, and each square centimeter treated with the required time to a tissue energy dose of 2 J/cm²)	II	Patients receiving HSCT conditioned with high-dose chemotherapy, with or without total body irradiation	Cancer of any kind
Benzydamine mouthwash	I	Patients receiving moderate-dose radiation therapy (up to 50 Gy) without concomitant chemotherapy	Head and neck cancer
KGF-1/palifermin (recombinant human keratinocyte growth factor-1) at a dose of 60 µg/kg per day for 3 days before conditioning treatment and for 3 days after transplant	II	• **Original MASCC/ISOO guideline**: Patients receiving high-dose chemotherapy and total body irradiation (TBI), followed by autologous stem cell transplantation • **Updated ESMO guideline**: Patients receiving chemotherapy and/or targeted agents, and/or HSCT with or without total body irradiation (local–regional radiotherapy alone not included), and who are anticipated to develop grade 3 or grade 4 oral mucositis	Hematological malignancy

Recommendation Against an Intervention	Level of Evidence	Therapy	Cancer
Glutamine i.v.	II	Patients receiving high-dose chemotherapy, with or without total body irradiation, for HSCT	Cancer of any kind
Iseganan antimicrobial mouthwash	II	Patients receiving high-dose chemotherapy, with or without total body irradiation, for HSCT	Cancer of any kind
Sucralfate mouthwash	I	Patients receiving chemotherapy for cancer	Cancer of any kind
PTA (polymyxin, tobramycin, amphotericin B) paste and BCoG antimicrobial lozenges	II	Patients receiving radiation therapy without concomitant chemotherapy	Head and neck cancer
Iseganan antimicrobial mouthwash	II	Patients receiving radiation therapy or concomitant chemoradiation for head and neck cancer	Head and neck cancer
Sucralfate mouthwash	I II	Patients receiving radiation therapy or concomitant chemoradiation	Head and neck cancer

Source: Peterson DE et al. *Ann Oncol* 2015;26 Suppl 5:v139–51.

Note: Level of evidence used in the MASCC/ISOO guidelines (16,17).

Level I: Evidence obtained from meta-analysis of multiple, well-designed, controlled studies; randomized trials with low false-positive and false-negative errors (high power).

Level II: Evidence obtained from at least one well-designed experimental study; randomized trials with high false-positive and/or false-negative errors (low power).

Level III: Evidence obtained from well-designed, quasi-experimental studies such as nonrandomized, controlled single-group, pretest–posttest comparison, cohort, time, or matched case–control series.

Level IV: Evidence obtained from well-designed, nonexperimental studies, such as comparative and correlational descriptive and case studies.

Level V: Evidence obtained from case reports and clinical examples.

TABLE 8.5

Suggestions for Prevention of Oral Mucositis

Suggestion in Favor of an Intervention	Level of Evidence	Therapy	Cancer
Oral care protocols	III	All cancer treatment modalities	Cancer of any kind
Photobiomodulation (low-level laser therapy; wavelength around 632.8 nm)	III	Patients undergoing radiotherapy, without concomitant chemotherapy	Head and neck cancer
Oral cryotherapy	III	Patients receiving high-dose melphalan, with or without total body irradiation, as conditioning for HSCT	Hematological malignancy
Zinc supplements	III	Patients receiving radiation therapy or chemoradiation	Oral cancer

Suggestion Against an Intervention	Level of Evidence	Therapy	Cancer
GM-CSF (granulocyte–macrophage colony-stimulating factor) mouthwash	II	Patients receiving high-dose chemotherapy, for autologous or allogeneic stem cell transplantation	Cancer of any kind
Systemic pilocarpine	II	Patients receiving high-dose chemotherapy, with or without total body irradiation, for HSCT	Cancer of any kind
	III	Patients receiving radiation therapy	Head and neck cancer
Chlorhexidine mouthwash	III	Patients receiving radiation therapy	Head and neck cancer
Misoprostol mouthwash	III	Patients receiving radiation therapy	Head and neck cancer

Source: Peterson DE et al. *Ann Oncol* 2015;26 Suppl 5:v139–51.

Note: Level of evidence used in the MASCC/ISOO guidelines (16,17).

Level I: Evidence obtained from meta-analysis of multiple, well-designed, controlled studies; randomized trials with low false-positive and false-negative errors (high power).

Level II: Evidence obtained from at least one well-designed experimental study; randomized trials with high false-positive and/or false-negative errors (low power).

Level III: Evidence obtained from well-designed, quasi-experimental studies such as nonrandomized, controlled single-group, pretest–posttest comparison, cohort, time, or matched case–control series.

Level IV: Evidence obtained from well-designed, nonexperimental studies, such as comparative and correlational descriptive and case studies.

Level V: Evidence obtained from case reports and clinical examples.

Pigmentary Changes

Hyperpigmentation is a well-recognized complication of cancer chemotherapeutic agents. The skin (postinflammatory hyperpigmentation, flagellate or reticulate dermatitis, "diffuse tan," supravenous serpentine hyperpigmentation, eruptive nevi, etc.), nails (melanonychia striata, transverse or total melanonychia; Figure 8.3a), and the oral mucosal membranes may be affected. Although the pathogenesis remains to be determined, hyperpigmentation is thought to be secondary to a direct toxic effect of chemotherapy on melanocytes, stimulating melanin production (21,22).

Oral mucosal pigmentary changes can occur with a wide range of chemotherapeutic agents (21,22), notably, busulfan, bleomycin, cyclophosphamide, cisplatin, 5-fluorouracil, doxorubicin, tegafur, daunorubicin, hydroxyurea, and capecitabine. Because the lesions are asymptomatic, the overall incidence probably remains underestimated. Black to brownish lesions can occur locally or more diffusely, and can involve both keratinized and nonkeratinized mucosae (patchy, linear, or diffuse hyperpigmented macules on the lips [Figure 8.3b]; the ventral or dorsal aspect of the tongue [Figure 8.3c], gingiva, oral mucosa, or the palate). They can develop in an isolated manner, or in association with skin hyperpigmentation or melanonychia (21,22).

Chemo-induced mucosal hyperpigmentation often persists for months after treatment discontinuation, but a gradual fading is usually noted, with complete disappearance in some cases (Figure 8.3d).

TABLE 8.6

Recommendations and Suggestions for Treatment of Oral Mucositis

Recommendation in Favor of an Intervention	Level of Evidence	Therapy	Cancer
Morphine (patient-controlled analgesia)	II	Patients undergoing HSCT	Cancer of any kind
Recommendation Against an Intervention	**Level of Evidence**	**Therapy**	**Cancer**
Sucralfate mouthwash	II	Patients receiving radiation therapy	Cancer of any kind
Suggestion in Favor of an Intervention	**Level of Evidence**	**Therapy**	**Cancer**
Doxepin mouthwash (0.5%) (to control pain due to mucositis)	IV	All cancer treatment modalities	Cancer of any kind
Transdermal fentanyl (to control pain due to mucositis)	III	Patients receiving conventional and high-dose chemotherapy, with or without total body irradiation	Cancer of any kind
Morphine mouthwash (0.2%) (to control pain due to mucositis)	III	Patients receiving chemoradiation therapy	Head and neck cancer

Source: Peterson DE et al. *Ann Oncol* 2015;26 Suppl 5:v139–51.

Note: Level of evidence used in the MASCC/ISOO guidelines (16,17).

Level I: Evidence obtained from meta-analysis of multiple, well-designed, controlled studies; randomized trials with low false-positive and false-negative errors (high power).

Level II: Evidence obtained from at least one well-designed experimental study; randomized trials with high false-positive and/or false-negative errors (low power).

Level III: Evidence obtained from well-designed, quasi-experimental studies such as nonrandomized, controlled single-group, pretest–posttest comparison, cohort, time, or matched case–control series.

Level IV: Evidence obtained from well-designed, nonexperimental studies, such as comparative and correlational descriptive and case studies.

Level V: Evidence obtained from case reports and clinical examples.

No specific management is required and patients only need reassurance. A prospective follow-up, however, should be proposed (21,22).

Taste Alterations

According to some estimates, 50% of patients treated with chemotherapy alone and about 75% of patients treated by both chemotherapy and head and neck radiation therapy experience taste alterations (13,23). A statistically significant correlation exists between the type of chemotherapy and the occurrence of dysgeusia (24). The burden of taste alteration can be at the forefront of complaints related to some chemotherapeutic agents (taxane, 5-fluorouracil, melphalan, busulfan, thiotepa, etoposide, cyclophosphamide, etc.) or combination of drugs (R-CHOP, TPF, FEC regimens, etc.) and can result in poor eating behavior (25). Suggestions of interventions for management are listed in Tables 8.3 and 8.7.

Xerostomia

Chemotherapeutic drugs can induce temporary (but sometimes impairing) xerostomia, associated with burning mouth and soreness. This condition is preceded by a metallic taste in some cases, enhancing the sensation of dysgeusia (13,14). It generally disappears during the year following the end of chemotherapeutic treatment. Supportive care measures should be delivered (Tables 8.3 and 8.7). Moreover, dental hypersensitivity is not rare in this context, and daily application of fluoride gel with a gum shield should be considered as a symptomatic measure and for the prevention of dental caries (4).

TABLE 8.7

Main Interventions for Management of Mucosal Changes Induced by Anticancer Therapies

Mucosal Changes	Main Interventions for Management
Mucositis/stomatitis/ aphthous-like lesions	See also Tables 8.3, 8.4, 8.5, 8.6, and 8.8 To discuss: steroids (topical, intralesional, oral), morphine mouthwash, systemic analgesics, photobiomodulation Dose modifications (to be discussed with the oncologist) Offset of radiotherapy sessions (to be discussed with the radiotherapist)
Xerostomia	Basic oral care/dietary recommendations (Table 8.3) Hydration, sugar-free gum or candy stimulants; sialogogues: pilocarpine, anethole trithione, cevimeline, bethanechol; artificial saliva substitutes (palliation); thermal water; frequent sips of water
Taste alterations	Basic oral care/dietary recommendations (Table 8.3) Dose modification or changes to medication (to be discussed with the oncologist)
Pigmentary changes	No specific local interventions; regular follow-up and biopsy in case of atypical lesions
Oral lichenoid reactions	Topical corticosteroids (clobetasol propionate) for painful lesions; regular oral examinations with long-term follow-up
Dysesthesia	Basic oral care/dietary recommendations (Table 8.3) Avoidance of irritating foods and symptomatic relief through topical analgesics Medications for neuropathy (clonazepam, gabapentin, antidepressants)
Benign migratory glossitis	No specific local interventions; avoidance of irritating foods; steroid mouth rinse three times per day for a few days or tacrolimus cream (0.1%) for painful lesions
Hyperkeratotic lesions; gingival hyperplasia	No specific local interventions; monthly examination and biopsy in case of atypical lesions
Telangiectasia/mucosal bleeding/delayed healing	Basic oral care (Table 8.3) Dose modifications (to be discussed with the oncologist)

Source: Vigarios E et al. *Support Care Cancer* 2017;25:1713–39.

Mucosal Bleeding

Spontaneous or induced hemorrhage can occur with myelosuppression (platelet counts below 20,000 cells/ mm^3). Mucosal bleeding usually appears after local trauma, especially in patients with preexisting periodontal disease (13,14). Gingival bleeding is the most common manifestation. Petechiae, ecchymoses, or hematomas can also be observed.

Head and Neck Radiation Therapy

Oral Mucositis

Oral mucositis may develop in nearly all patients undergoing radiotherapy for head and neck cancer (1,8,10–12,18,26–28). Lesions occur in the first 2 to 3 weeks in the form of painful hyperemia/erythema, and progress to ulcerations with fibrin-exudate pseudomembranes, which usually appear at more than 30 grays. They are strictly confined to within the irradiated field and may involve any radiation-exposed (nonkeratinized and keratinized) oral tissues (Figure 8.4a through e). Radio-induced oral mucositis represents the most distressing and disabling acute toxicity in head and neck cancer patients. Oral pain may lead to significant functional impairment and may severely impact oral function and nutritional intake. Patients also report swallowing difficulties, dysgeusia, dysphagia, xerostomia, and speech difficulties, all of which contribute to morbidity and have negative effects on patients' quality of life. Septic complications may also occur (herpes simplex reactivation, oropharyngeal candidiasis, bacterial infections), which further aggravate the symptoms and may induce systemic infection. Oral infection should be systematically considered in any case with an atypical or severe presentation, and for mucosal lesions extending beyond the irradiated area.

Poor oral health and hygiene, age older than 65 years, gender (increased risk in females), concomitant periodontal disease, salivary gland dysfunction, inadequate nutritional status, tumor location, genomic

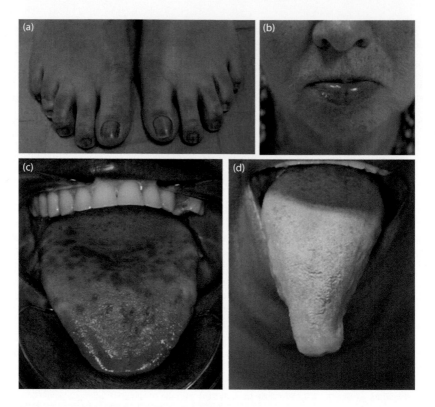

FIGURE 8.3   Chemo-induced pigmentary changes. (a) Multiple melanonychia striata, involving all toenails (hydroxyurea). (b) Linear hyperpigmented macules on the lips (capecitabine). (c) Hyperpigmentation of the dorsum of the tongue induced by chemotherapy (capecitabine). (d) Clinical presentation of the same patient 18 months after chemotherapy discontinuation. Note a complete disappearance of the lesions.

factors, smoking, local trauma, and underlying comorbidities (e.g., diabetes mellitus, impaired renal function) represent aggravating factors. In addition, oral mucositis is usually more frequent, more extensive, and more severe in head and neck cancer patients treated concomitantly with chemotherapy (e.g., cisplatin) and/or targeted therapy (e.g., anti-EGFR; see also section "Mucositis"). The overall incidence is higher when the total radiation dose used is increased and when altered fractionation radiotherapy is used rather than conventional fractionated radiotherapy. Three-dimensional conformal radiotherapy techniques and intensity-modulated radiation therapy (IMRT) may allow a relative sparing of healthy oral tissues to peritumoral doses of radiation.

Proactive supportive management is paramount for these patients, as radiotherapy interruption or radiation dose limitation may compromise local tumor control and patient survival through repopulation of resistant clonal cells. Management potentially includes the use of opioid-derived analgesics, a gastrostomy tube or parenteral feeding, and hospitalization if needed. Lesions are transient and usually resolve within 3 to 8 weeks after stopping radiotherapy. However, persistent or recurrent forms have been identified recently, with chronic atrophy, erythema, and/or ulcers (29–31).

Management of radio-induced mucositis relies on the same protocols as those previously described for mucositis induced by chemotherapy (Tables 8.3 through 8.7).

Chronic Toxicities and Sequelae

Xerostomia

Xerostomia is the most common and prominent oral toxicity reported following head and neck radiation therapy (26,32–34). Definitive damage may occur to the major (parotid and submandibular) and minor

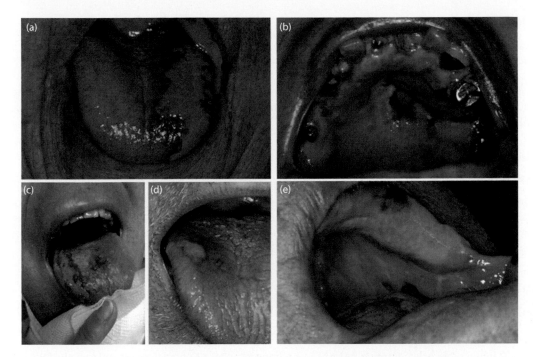

FIGURE 8.4 Radio-induced mucositis. (a) High-grade mucositis involving the half-side of the dorsum of the tongue (keratinized mucosa). (b) Poorly circumscribed mucositis involving the hard palate (keratinized mucosa). (c) Grade 3/4 mucositis of the lateral and dorsal aspects of the tongue (keratinized and nonkeratinized mucosae). (d) Limited lesions on the dorsum of the tongue (keratinized mucosa). (e) Very extensive mucositis within the field of irradiation, involving both keratinized and nonkeratinized mucosae (buccal mucosa, labial mucosa, and the dorsal aspect of the tongue).

salivary glands. Salivary gland hypofunction may result in permanent xerostomia. Saliva becomes scant, sticky, and viscous. The patient may also experience oral discomfort and pain. Furthermore, chronic xerostomia may increase the risk of oral infections or dental caries, and can lead to difficulties in speech, chewing, and swallowing, which significantly impact patients' quality of life.

Supportive care measures should be delivered systematically (Tables 8.3 and 8.7). Treatment essentially relies upon stimulation of the residual secretory capacity of the salivary glands with cholinergic agonists (such as pilocarpine or cevimeline), which have been shown to reduce xerostomia and increase salivary flow rate compared to placebo (32–34). In addition, it has been reported that the concomitant administration of pilocarpine during radiotherapy could also increase the unstimulated salivary flow rate and may be of short-term benefit (34). Saliva substitute solutions might be also useful. Daily application of topical fluoride gel is mandatory to limit dental damage secondary to persistent saliva changes.

Finally, it is fundamental to note that IMRT, which allows accurate delineation of the tumor volume and the relative preservation of organs at risk (e.g., the parotid gland), is associated with a lower incidence of severe postradiation xerostomia (26).

Taste Alterations

Two-thirds of patients treated with head and neck radiotherapy experience taste alterations. All five primary taste qualities are affected (23). Radiation may directly modify smell and taste sensations, but these alterations can be also related to xerostomia. Persistent taste loss may be caused by damage to taste receptors or C-/A-delta fibers, and by salivary flow modifications (23,27). Recovery from dysgeusia is variable; improvement is usually observed in 2–6 months following radiotherapy, but symptoms may become permanent in some cases (23). Modulated radiation therapy that spares the parotid glands allows recovery of salivary secretions, as well as of taste function (23,26). Management includes patient education with dietary counseling (Tables 8.3 and 8.7).

Other Sequelae

Radiotherapy may result in progressive deterioration of dental and periodontal tissues, which leads to an increased risk of caries and periodontitis. Hyposalivation also promotes the development of dental caries ("radiation caries") (27).

Postradiation fibrosis (including trismus) and osteoradionecrosis may also occur, but the reported incidence of these toxicities has significantly decreased with modern radiotherapy delivery techniques (3D radiotherapy and IMRT) (27).

Targeted Therapies

Oral toxicities of targeted therapies may display very characteristic features, which clearly differ from the classic oral injuries observed with cytotoxic chemotherapy and/or radiotherapy (Table 8.1). Targeted therapy-related oral toxicities frequently affect more than 20% of treated patients and can lead to significant morbidity or treatment interruption (4,12,16,35–42).

mTOR Inhibitors

mTOR Inhibitor-Associated Stomatitis

Incidence

mTOR inhibitor-associated stomatitis (mIAS) is a frequent and well-characterized oral toxicity, for which meta-analyses indicate that the overall incidence of any grade and high grade (≥ 3, following NCI-CTCae V4.02) mIAS range from 33.5 to 52.9% and from 4.1 to 5.4%, respectively, regardless of the type of mTOR inhibitor therapy (everolimus, temsirolimus) (44,45,49) (Table 8.1). It mostly occurs within the first cycle of treatment (44–46) and should be considered as a class effect. mIAS represents the most prevalent adverse event associated with mTOR therapy and the most frequent dose-limiting toxicity (4,44). In addition, the therapeutic use of everolimus in combination with endocrine agents (exemestane) in breast cancer has been associated with significant increases in the all-grade incidence of mIAS (47), with more than two-thirds of patients being affected.

Clinical Presentation

mIAS is characterized by single or multiple, painful, and well-circumscribed round/ovoid superficial ulcers (aphthous-like stomatitis), mainly developing on the nonkeratinized mucosa (4,35,38,43,44,48,49). The lesions generally measure a few millimeters in diameter and display a central gray area that is surrounded by a perilesional erythematous halo, mimicking recurrent aphthous stomatitis or herpetic lesions (Figure 8.5a through d). In contrast to chemo-induced mucositis, mIAS typically spares other mucosae.

Management

Preventive management consists of the promotion of good oral hygiene, relying on basic oral care recommendations (Table 8.3). Pretherapeutic oral screening is recommended in order to identify potential sources of trauma and dental or periodontal disease outbreaks. In a recent phase II prevention trial (SWISH trial) (50), the prophylactic use of dexamethasone mouthwash (0.5 mg/5 mL, 4 times daily for 8 weeks) in patients receiving everolimus (10 mg) and exemestane (25 mg) for advanced or metastatic breast cancer significantly reduced the all-grade incidence of mIAS (21.2% all-grade incidence, grade ≥ 2 below 3% without any grade 3; indirect comparison).

In accordance with the latest ESMO clinical practice guidelines (16), corticosteroids should be recommended as the first-line treatment for mIAS: mostly topical steroids (steroid mouthwash [e.g., dexamethasone mouthwash, 0.1 mg/mL] or topical application of high-potency corticosteroids [clobetasol 0.05% gel or cream]), with use of intralesional or systemic corticosteroids if needed. In our experience, this "steroid regimen" can be associated with photobiomodulation (low-level laser therapy: wavelength of 633–685 or 780–830 nm; power output of between 10 and 150 mW; energy density 2–3 J/

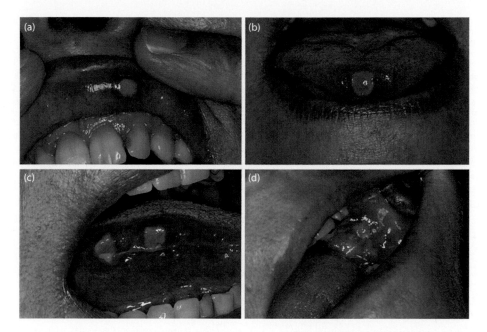

FIGURE 8.5 mTOR inhibitors. (a,b) Typical mIAS induced by everolimus, with an erythematous halo (lesions exclusively involving the nonkeratinized mucosa). (c,d) Multiple aphthous-like lesions in patients treated with everolimus and exemestane in combination.

cm^2 and no more than 6 J/cm^2 on the tissue surface treated) (4). High-grade mIAS may also be managed by dose adjustments (Table 8.8). As an example, dose modifications and treatment discontinuation were required in about 5% and 2% of treated patients in main clinical trials, respectively (44,46,48,49). The severity and/or the recurrence of the lesions, as well as the time needed to recover, will determine whether full dosing can be resumed or whether dose reduction or discontinuation is required (4,39,47).

Taste Alterations

Dysgeusia has been reported in up to one-third of everolimus-treated patients (4), but probably remains underreported (23,51). No dose adjustment is usually required. Due to the lack of standardized preventive and curative treatment, management (Tables 8.3 and 8.7) relies on symptomatic dietary support.

Xerostomia

Mild xerostomia has been sporadically reported in everolimus-treated patients (about 6%) (4).

HER Inhibitors

The HER inhibitor therapeutic family includes monoclonal antibodies (cetuximab, panitumumab) and tyrosine kinase inhibitors (gefitinib, erlotinib) targeting the EGF receptor (epidermal growth factor receptor, HER1), as well as multitargeted kinase inhibitors (afatinib, lapatinib, and dacomitinib) inhibiting both EGFR and other HER (or ErbB) receptors (Table 8.1) (4,35,52–58).

Mucositis

Incidence

- *EGFR/HER1 tyrosine kinase inhibitors*: The all-grade incidence of mucositis induced by erlotinib and gefitinib used in monotherapy varies between 8 and 20% and 19 and 24%, respectively (4). Moreover, the incidence rate of high-grade ($\geq$3) mucositis has never been reported to exceed 1%, with neither erlotinib nor gefitinib.

TABLE 8.8

Modified Management Algorithm for mIAS Induced by mTOR Inhibitors

Grade 1[a] Erythema of Mucosa with Asymptomatic or Mild Symptoms	Grade 2 Patchy Ulceration with Moderate Pain; No Interference with Oral Intake	Grade 3 Confluent Ulcerations or Pseudomembranes with Severe Pain, Interfering with Oral Intake

Supportive care: Basic oral care[b] and symptomatic management in case of mild symptoms (corticosteroid mouthwash)
No dietary modifications
Continue mTOR inhibitor
Monitor for change in severity
	Symptomatic management and supportive care: Basic oral care,[b] topical steroids, photobiomodulation (LLLT), modified diet
	Dose adjustment:
	• If toxicity is tolerable
	    • No dose adjustment required
	• If toxicity becomes intolerable
	    • Temporary dose interruption until recovery to grade ≤1
	    • Reinitiate treatment at same dose
	• If toxicity recurs at grade 2
	    • Manage as first grade 3 flare: interrupt treatment until recovery to grade ≤1
	    • Reinitiate at a lower dose (i.e., 5 mg/day for everolimus)
	Monitor for change in severity
		Symptomatic management and supportive care: basic oral care,[b] systemic corticosteroids, photobiomodulation, morphine mouthwash, modified diet, systemic analgesics
		Dose adjustment:
		• Temporary dose interruption until recovery to grade ≤1; reinitiate treatment at a lower dose
		• If toxicity recurs at grade 3
		    • Manage as grade 4; consider discontinuation
		Monitor for change in severity

Source: Vigarios E et al. *Support Care Cancer* 2017;25:1713–39. With permission.
[a] Grade refers to NCI CTCAE v4.0.
[b] Basic oral care, see Table 8.3.

- *Pan-HER tyrosine kinase inhibitors*: Conversely, with the new generation of pan-HER tyrosine kinase inhibitors, mucositis appears to be one of the main toxicities, after paronychia, diarrhea, and papulopustular rash (52). The incidence of all-grade mucositis induced by afatinib appears to be significantly higher than that of erlotinib or gefitinib, and ranges from 29 to 64%. All-grade incidence reported with dacomitinib appears to be very similar to afatinib (about 40%). Finally, high-grade (≥3) mucositis induced by afatinib and dacomitinib may occur in 3–7% of treated patients (4).

- *Monoclonal antibodies targeting EGFR*: Mucositis appears to occur less frequently with cetuximab or panitumumab monotherapy than with tyrosine kinase inhibitors (53). In one comparative phase III study, the incidence of all-grade mucositis was 7% in patients treated with cetuximab and 5% in those treated with panitumumab (<1% of grade 3 in both groups).

- *Cetuximab or panitumumab in combination with chemotherapy*: Cetuximab and panitumumab are seldom used as monotherapies, and are usually combined with chemotherapeutic regimens and/or radiation therapy. Cetuximab and panitumumab when combined with chemotherapy both significantly increase the risk of developing mucositis of any grade compared to chemotherapy alone (54).

- *Cetuximab in association with head and neck radiation therapy*: The incidence of high-grade (≥3) mucositis is also high when cetuximab is combined with radiation therapy, particularly when being used for the treatment of advanced head and neck cancers (about 60%) (55). The main pivotal studies, however, initially reported that the addition of cetuximab to radiotherapy didn't have a significant impact on the incidence of high-grade (≥3) mucositis in comparison to radiotherapy alone. However, our experience and that of other authors (56) indicates that a higher incidence of severe mucositis is commonly observed with this therapeutic combination. The same tendency is observed when combining cetuximab with head and neck radiochemotherapy versus head and neck radiochemotherapy without cetuximab. Finally, the incidence of high-grade (≥3) mucositis also seems to be higher when cetuximab is used in combination with radiotherapy than when chemotherapy is used in combination with radiation therapy in head and neck cancer (4).

Clinical Presentation

Clinically, mucositis corresponds to a moderate erythema, sometimes associated with limited and superficial ulcers occurring shortly after treatment introduction (4,35,56,57). It can take on the appearance of aphthous-like lesions (Figure 8.6a through c), although these lesions are less typical than those described previously with mTOR inhibitors. All nonkeratinized areas may be involved. Of note, lip lesions are quite common, including erythema, erosions, cracks (52), and angular cheilitis (58).

The addition of cetuximab to head and neck radiation therapy for the management of locally advanced squamous cell carcinoma is associated with severe lesions involving both nonkeratinized and keratinized areas (Figure 8.6d). These lesions are frequently multiple and polycyclic, and often associated with significant functional impairment and perioral radiodermatitis. Interestingly, patients may present with mucosal pain, although mucosal changes remain limited. The association of monoclonal antibodies targeting EGFR with chemotherapy is also associated with more severe mucosal involvement (Figure 8.6e).

Management

Recommendations for preventive and curative management of mucositis induced by HER inhibitors are similar to those previously described for mIAS (Tables 8.3 and 8.7). Dose adjustments and offset of any radiation therapy sessions is sometimes required and should be discussed in close collaboration with the referent oncologist/radiotherapist.

Other Oral Toxicities

Dysgeusia and xerostomia are mainly reported with new generation HER tyrosine kinase inhibitors (dacomitinib, afatinib) and are mostly of mild intensity, requiring no specific management (4).

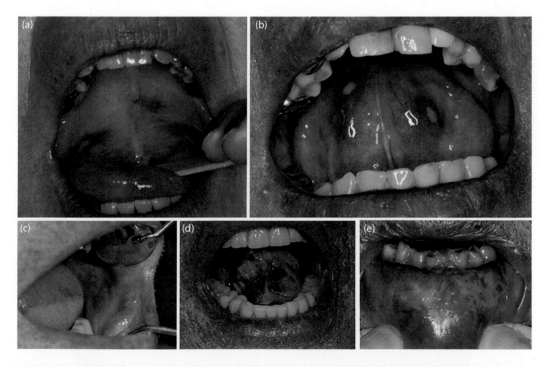

FIGURE 8.6 HER inhibitors. (a) Superficial ulcers induced by the pan-HER inhibitor afatinib, involving the nonkeratinized mucosa (soft palate). (b) Mucositis with well-circumscribed aphthous-like lesions on the ventral side of the tongue (erlotinib). (c) Limited mucositis of the buccal mucosa induced by cetuximab monotherapy. (d) Grade 3 mucositis with the combination of cetuximab and head and neck radiation therapy (see associated perioral radiodermatitis). (e) Diffuse mucositis of the labial mucosa observed with treatment combining panitumumab and chemotherapy (carboplatin, 5FU, cetuximab).

Angiogenesis Inhibitors

The angiogenesis inhibitor class of targeted therapies includes monoclonal antibodies (bevacizumab, ramucirumab) that directly inhibit the vascular endothelial growth factor and multikinase inhibitors (sunitinib, sorafenib, pazopanib, axitinib, cabozantinib) targeting the angiogenic receptors (VEGF receptor [VEGFR], platelet-derived growth factor receptor [PDGFR]) and other distinct signaling pathways (Table 8.1) (4,35,37,38,53,59–65).

Stomatitis

Incidence

About 25% of patients treated with multitargeted angiogenesis inhibitors develop stomatitis within the first 2 months of therapy (4,37,59). In the main pivotal studies, the incidence of all grades of stomatitis induced by angiogenesis inhibitors ranges from 7 to 29%, depending on the drug used. However, stomatitis is clearly more frequent with sunitinib, sorafenib, or the newly registered cabozantinib. Comparative studies underline that the incidence of all-grade angiogenesis inhibitor–associated stomatitis is lower than that of all-grade mIAS (38,60).

With sunitinib, stomatitis appears to be one of the most frequent adverse events (after diarrhea, fatigue, and nausea), with an any-grade incidence ranging from 22 to 27% (61). The latter appears to be higher than that of stomatitis associated with other first-generation multitargeted angiogenesis inhibitors, in particular sorafenib, for which the incidence of all-grade stomatitis is reported to range from 7 to 19% (4). On the other hand, the incidence of all-grade stomatitis with cabozantinib is similar to that reported with sunitinib, having been reported in 22–29% of treated patients (60).

The incidence of high-grade ($\geq$3) stomatitis has never been reported to exceed 4% with any multitargeted angiogenesis inhibitor (60,61) (Table 8.1).

Clinical Presentation

The broad term "stomatitis" has been used to describe a range of mucosal injuries or toxicities (such as mucosal sensitivity, taste alterations, dry mouth, and oral ulcerations) associated with angiogenesis inhibitors (12,37). However, oral changes observed with multitargeted angiogenesis inhibitors mainly correspond to a diffuse mucosal hypersensitivity/dysesthesia (37), in some cases associated with moderate erythema (38) (Figure 8.7a) or painful inflammation of the oral mucosa (including a burning mouth, discomfort induced by hot or spicy foods) (37). Less frequently, well-limited ulcerations (Figure 8.7b) or

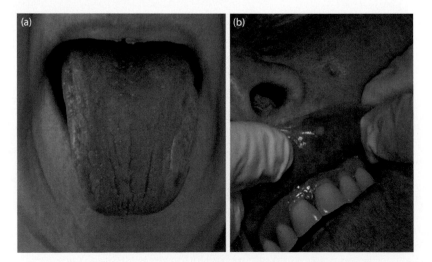

FIGURE 8.7 Angiogenesis inhibitors. (a) Typical clinical presentation in a cabozantinib-treated patient reporting dysesthesia. (b) Isolated aphthous-like ulceration observed with the multikinase angiogenesis inhibitor sunitinib.

linear ulcers of the nonkeratinized mucosa may also be reported, particularly with sunitinib or sorafenib (4,35,59). Rapid onset after treatment initiation (first weeks of treatment) and gradual disappearance is generally noted (37,38,62).

Management of mucosal hypersensitivity relies on the same interventions as those described for mIAS or mucositis induced by EGFR inhibitors, associated with dietary measures (4) (Tables 8.4 through 8.7). Dose adjustment (<10% of treated patients) or treatment discontinuation (about 1% of treated patients) (37,59), however, are only rarely needed.

Taste Alterations

Taste changes appear to be the second most frequent oral adverse event (37) induced by multitargeted antiangiogenic kinase inhibitors. They are most often reported with sunitinib and cabozantinib, for which the incidence of all grades of dysgeusia ranges from 20 to 49% and 24 to 34% of treated patients (60), respectively. High-grade dysgeusia is clearly uncommon, occurring in less than 1% of treated patients. However, comparative studies indicate that dysgeusia is more common in patients treated with angiogenesis inhibitors than in those treated with mTOR inhibitors (4).

Suggested therapeutic options for management are described in Tables 8.3 and 8.7.

Benign Migratory Glossitis

Induced benign migratory glossitis can be observed with both monoclonal antibody bevacizumab (Figure 8.8a) and multikinase angiogenesis inhibitors (sunitinib [Figure 8.8b], sorafenib, axitinib, etc.). Specific management is usually not required and patients only need reassurance (Table 8.7). Progressive disappearance of the lesions is generally noted in a few months after treatment discontinuation (63,64).

Other Oral Toxicities

Depending on the series, 4–12% of patients treated with multitargeted angiogenesis inhibitors develop grade 1–2 xerostomia (4). Bleeding events and delayed wound healing can be also associated with these drugs and should be systematically taken into consideration before oral surgery.

Typical yellow oral mucosal discoloration and localized hyperkeratotic lesions have been sporadically reported with sunitinib and the pan-RAF inhibitor sorafenib (Figure 8.9), respectively.

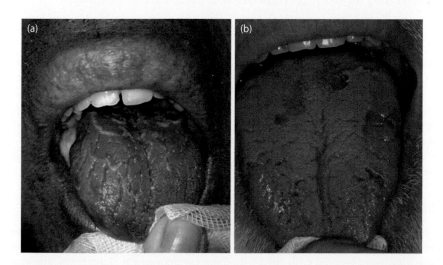

FIGURE 8.8 Angiogenesis inhibitors. Benign migratory glossitis induced by (a) bevacizumab and (b) sunitinib.

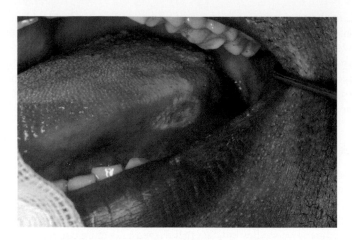

FIGURE 8.9   Localized hyperkeratotic lesion with the multikinase angiogenesis inhibitor sorafenib (with pan-RAF inhibitory activity).

The association of antiresorptive drugs (bisphosphonates, e.g., zoledronic acid, pamidronate, and the inhibitor of RANKL [receptor activator of nuclear factor κB ligand] [denosumab]) with antiangiogenic targeted therapies (sunitinib, bevacizumab) significantly increases the risk of developing medication-related osteonecrosis of the jaw (65), most often after oral surgery (Tables 8.1 and 8.7).

BCR-ABL Inhibitor: Imatinib

Oral Lichenoid Reactions

The development of oral lichenoid reactions (Figure 8.10) with imatinib is the most frequently individualized oral adverse event with this drug (Table 8.1) (66–69). Systematic screening for concomitant nail or cutaneous involvement should be also performed. Lesions are usually polymorphic, combining reticular streaks together with whitish papules, erosion, or atrophy. They are mainly located on the buccal or lingual mucosa. These lesions gradually develop after several months of treatment and frequently remain asymptomatic. Therefore, a systematic examination of the oral cavity is required in patients treated with imatinib (Table 8.7). No dose modification is generally needed. However, a prospective follow-up is mandatory because of the potential risk of malignant transformation.

Pigmentary Changes

A fairly typical "blue-gray" asymptomatic hyperpigmentation of the hard palate may be noted in patients treated with imatinib (Figure 8.11) (70,71). Oral hyperpigmentation in other locations has been described in anecdotal reports (71). The pathophysiological mechanism seems similar to that of hyperpigmentation due to antimalarials (drug metabolite deposition in the mucosa and complex formation with hemosiderin or melanin). Direct inhibition of c-kit (which is physiologically expressed in the oral mucosa) by imatinib has been also implicated in this mechanism by some authors.

To our knowledge, these oral changes have not been described until now with new generation BCR-ABL inhibitors (nilotinib, dasatinib, ponatinib).

BRAF Inhibitors

Induced cutaneous hyperkeratotic lesions (e.g., verrucous papilloma, hand foot skin reaction, keratosis pilaris–like rash, keratoacanthoma, and squamous cell carcinoma) represent the most common dermatologic toxicities observed with BRAF inhibitors (vemurafenib, dabrafenib, encorafenib) when prescribed in monotherapy (72) (Table 8.1) (72–74). Less frequently, multifocal asymptomatic mucosal

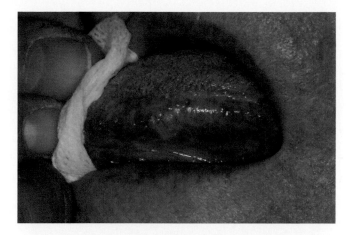

FIGURE 8.10 Typical lichenoid reaction with visible reticular streaks on the lateral side of the tongue (imatinib).

hyperkeratotic lesions have also been noted. These lesions are predominantly located on the linea alba, gingival margin (Figure 8.12), and hard palate. Malignant transformation of these oral hyperkeratotic lesions into squamous cell carcinoma is rare but possible (73) (Table 8.7). Therefore, a regular oral follow-up should be recommended in patients treated in monotherapy. However, BRAF inhibitors are now mostly used in combination with MEK inhibitors (vemurafenib–cobimetinib, dabrafenib–trametinib). By blocking the MAP kinase pathway downstream, MEK inhibitors significantly limit the development of secondary cutaneous or mucosal hyperkeratotic lesions.

Finally, gingival hyperplasia has been described anecdotally with vemurafenib (74).

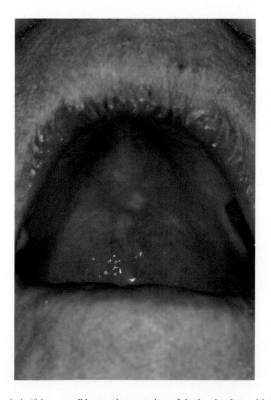

FIGURE 8.11 Fairly characteristic "blue-gray" hyperpigmentation of the hard palate with imatinib.

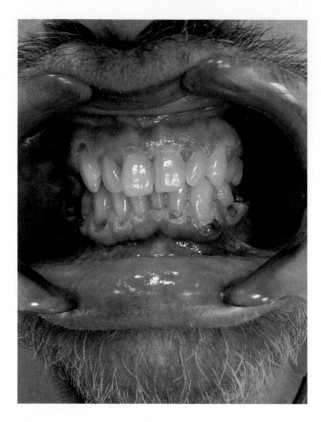

FIGURE 8.12   Hyperkeratotic lesions on the marginal gingiva with BRAF inhibitors (vemurafenib).

Selective Pan-FGFR Inhibitors

Xerostomia represents one of the most frequent treatment-emergent adverse events reported with the new selective pan-FGFR inhibitors (under development). It may affect between 20 and 45% of treated patients (75,76). In our experience, xerostomia is frequently of grade 3 (Figure 8.13) and can be very debilitating and severely impair a patient's quality of life (77). Xerophthalmia and skin xerosis are commonly associated (76). In addition, dysgeusia, hair changes with trichomegaly, and severe onycholysis are also usually noted with selective FGFR inhibitors (77).

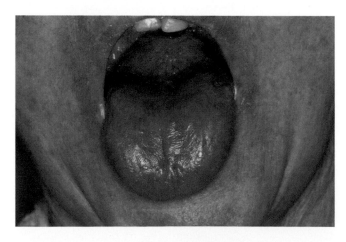

FIGURE 8.13   Grade 3 xerostomia induced by new selective pan-FGFR inhibitors.

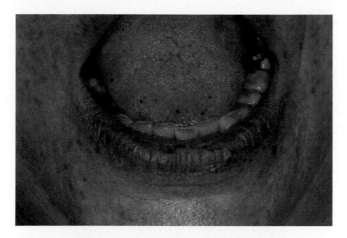

FIGURE 8.14   Multiple mucosal telangiectasias involving the lip and the tongue (TDM-1).

TDM-1 (Antibody-Drug Conjugate Ado-Trastuzumab Emtansine)

Cutaneous and mucosal telangiectasias, mimicking Osler-Weber-Rendu syndrome, have been observed with the antibody-drug conjugate ado-trastuzumab emtansine (TDM-1) (Table 8.1) (78,79). They appear as spider cutaneous telangiectasias and dome-shaped mucosal lesions with surrounding small radiating dilated vessels (Figure 8.14). Regular screening for mucosal telangiectasias is recommended in this context (Table 8.7).

ALK Inhibitors

A mild to moderate dysgeusia may be noted in 10–25% of patients treated with crizotinib. Finally, all-grade stomatitis (without any grade 3) is reported in about 15% of patients (Table 8.1) (80).

Hedgehog Pathway Inhibitors

Taste alteration is the most frequent reported toxicity with vismodegib, after muscle spasms. Depending on the series, 51–84% and 22% of treated patients developed grade 1–2 dysgeusia and ageusia, respectively (Table 8.1) (81,82). Treatment interruption is reported in about 5% of treated patients. Management (Tables 8.3 and 8.7) relies on proactive education of the patients, including nutritional counseling, maintenance of good oral health, and rigorous follow-up of the weight curve.

Immune Checkpoint Inhibitors

Oral changes induced by immune checkpoint inhibitors have received limited attention to date in clinical trials, even though a spectrum of associated oral adverse events has recently emerged (5–7,83–92). Use of immune checkpoint inhibitors targeting the programmed cell death receptor-1 (PD-1) (nivolumab, pembrolizumab) or its ligand (PD-L1) (atezolizumab, durvalumab, avelumab) has been found to be associated with nonspecific moderate stomatitis or oral mucosal inflammation in sporadic cases (7,85,86). Recently, more characteristic oral lesions have been described (5,6,87–92).

Xerostomia

Mild to moderate xerostomia has been reported in about 5% of patients treated with anti-PD-1/PD-L1 antibodies (83–85). However, severe grade 3 xerostomia (Figure 8.15) can be also observed in several cases.

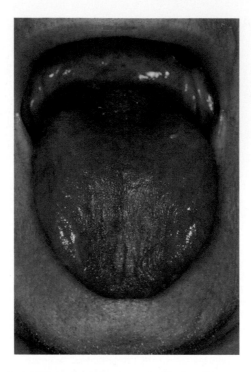

FIGURE 8.15   Immune checkpoint inhibitors. Grade 3 xerostomia (nivolumab).

Mucosal biopsies reveal histopathological features of a Gougerot-Sjögren–like syndrome, with cytotoxic T-cell (CD4+/CD8+) lymphocyte infiltration surrounding accessory salivary glands (Figure 8.16a through c). However, the detection of anti-SSA and anti-SSB antibodies is typically negative.

The occurrence—or worsening—of Goujerot-Sjögren syndrome has also been published sporadically with anti-PD-1 (together with arthralgias, sicca syndrome, and positivity of antinuclear and anti-SSA antibodies) (5).

Management relies on the supportive measures mentioned in Tables 8.3 and 8.7.

Dysgeusia

Moderate dysgeusia has been noted in less than 3% of PD-1– and PD-L1–treated patients. Xerostomia and dysgeusia appear less commonly with the anti-CTLA-4 agent, ipilimumab.

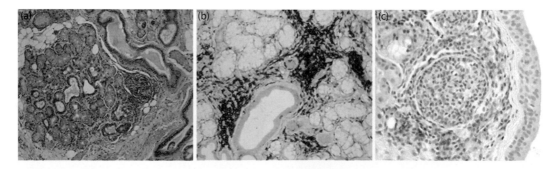

FIGURE 8.16   Immune checkpoint inhibitors. (a) Lymphohistiocytic infiltrate surrounding the salivary glands (HE, original magnification ×10). (b) Immunostaining revealing a predominantly CD4-positive T-cell infiltrate (original magnification ×20). (c) PD-L1 immunostaining (original magnification ×20). (Images courtesy of Dr. Colombat, IUCT France.)

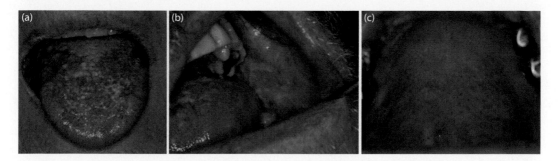

FIGURE 8.17 Immune checkpoint inhibitors. (a) Oral lichenoid reaction involving the dorsal aspect of the tongue (nivolumab). (b) Punctate and reticulated lichenoid lesions of the buccal mucosa and dorsum of the tongue (nivolumab). (c) Extensive reticulated lichenoid lesions developed on the palate (nivolumab).

Oral Lichenoid Reactions

Given their mechanism of action as immune-modulating agents that trigger T-cell activation, immune checkpoint inhibitors are associated with a specific toxicity profile, mostly of an immune mechanism-based nature (5,92). It is therefore not unusual to observe oral lichenoid reactions occurring several months after introduction of anti-PD1/PD-L1 therapy (5,90–92), strongly suggesting a class effect (92). Lesions most often occur in an isolated manner, but the skin, nails, or perianal/genital areas can be also involved simultaneously (5,91,92).

Oral examination reveals symmetric reticulated white streaks consistent with Wickham striae on the tongue (Figure 8.17a), buccal mucosa (Figure 8.17b), palate (Figure 8.17c), and mucosae of the inner lips/gingiva (92). Papular, plaque-like, ulcerative, or atrophic/erythematous lesions might also be observed, sometimes in combination. The keratinized and nonkeratinized mucosae can be affected. These induced lichenoid lesions usually remain self-limited and of low grade. Histologically, a moderate bandlike lymphohistiocytic infiltrate along the dermal epidermal junction is observed, together with patchy to florid vacuolar interface dermatitis; a partial disruption of the basal membrane zone; and apoptosis, hypergranulosis, and parakeratosis (92).

Oral lichenoid lesions have not been reported to lead to discontinuation or interruption of oncologic treatment, and, in most cases, they improved after several weeks of treatment with topical corticosteroids (clobetasol ointment or cream, dexamethasone/prednisolone mouthwash). Complete disappearance of the lesions after treatment discontinuation is generally observed (92). Regular follow-up is required regarding the potential risk of malignant transformation of lichenoid lesions (88,92) and a biopsy should be recommended for atypical lesions (Tables 8.3 and 8.7).

Other Toxicities

Anti-PD1 or anti-PD-L1 agents have been shown to result in a higher risk of developing immune-related bullous pemphigoid, sometimes involving the oral mucosa (5).

REFERENCES

1. Lalla RV, Saunders DP, Peterson DE. Chemotherapy or radiation-induced oral mucositis. *Dent Clin North Am* 2014;58:341–9.
2. Staudenmaier T et al. Burden of oral mucositis in stem cell transplant patients-the patients' perspective. *Support Care Cancer* Epub December 2, 2017.
3. Barkokebas A et al. Impact of oral mucositis on oral health-related quality of life of patients diagnosed with cancer. *J Oral Pathol Med* 2015;44:746–51.
4. Vigarios E, Epstein JB, Sibaud V. Oral mucosal changes induced by anticancer targeted therapies and immune checkpoint inhibitors. *Support Care Cancer* 2017;25:1713–39.

5. Sibaud V. Dermatologic reactions to immune checkpoint inhibitors: Skin toxicities and immunotherapy. *Am J Clin Dermatol* 2018;19:345–61.
6. Jackson LK et al. Oral health in oncology: Impact of immunotherapy. *Support Care Cancer* 2015;23:1–3.
7. Freeman-Keller M et al. Nivolumab in resected and unresecable metastatic melanoma: Characteristics of immune-related adverse events and association with outcomes. *Clin Cancer Res* 2016;22:886–94.
8. Peterson DE, Srivastava R, Lalla RV. Oral mucosal injury in oncology patients: Perspectives on maturation of a field. *Oral Dis* 2015;21:133–41.
9. Cinausero M et al. New frontiers in the pathobiology and treatment of cancer regimen-related mucosal injury. *Front Pharmacol* 2017;8:354.
10. Sonis ST. The pathobiology of mucositis. *Nat Rev Cancer* 2004;4:277–84.
11. Moslemi D et al. Management of chemo/radiation-induced oral mucositis in patients with head and neck cancer: A review of the current literature. *Radiother Oncol* 2016;120:13–20.
12. Al-Ansari S et al. Oral mucositis induced by anticancer therapies. *Curr Oral Health Rep* 2015;2:202–11.
13. Chaveli-López B. Oral toxicity produced by chemotherapy: A systematic review. *J Clin Exp Dent* 2014;6:e81–90.
14. Elad S, Zadik Y, Yarom N. Oral complications of nonsurgical cancer therapies. *Atlas Oral Maxillofac Surg Clin North Am* 2017;25:133–47.
15. Raber-Durlacher JE, Elad S, Barasch A. Oral mucositis. *Oral Oncol* 2010;46:452–6.
16. Peterson DE et al. Management of oral and gastrointestinal mucosal injury: ESMO Clinical Practice Guidelines for diagnosis, treatment, and follow-up. *Ann Oncol* 2015;26 Suppl 5:v139–51.
17. Lalla RV et al. Mucositis guidelines leadership group of the multinational association of supportive care in cancer and international society of oral oncology (MASCC/ISOO). MASCC/ISOO clinical practice guidelines for the management of mucositis secondary to cancer therapy. *Cancer* 2014;120:1453–61.
18. De Sanctis V et al. Mucositis in head and neck cancer patients treated with radiotherapy and systemic therapies: Literature review and consensus statements. *Crit Rev Oncol Hematol* 2016;100:147–66.
19. Elad S et al. Basic oral care for hematology-oncology patients and hematopoietic stem cell transplantation recipients: A position paper from the joint task force of the Multinational Association of Supportive Care in Cancer/International Society of Oral Oncology (MASCC/ISOO) and the European Society for Blood and Marrow Transplantation (EBMT). *Support Care Cancer* 2015;23:223–36.
20. Zecha JA et al. Low-level laser therapy/photobiomodulation in the management of side effects of chemoradiation therapy in head and neck cancer: Part 2: Proposed applications and treatment protocols. *Support Care Cancer* 2016;24:2793–805.
21. Bronner AK, Hood AF. Cutaneous complications of chemotherapeutic agents. *J Am Acad Dermatol* 1983;9:645–63.
22. Sibaud V et al. Pigmentary disorders induced by anticancer agents. Part I: Chemotherapy. *Ann Dermatol Venereol* 2013;140:183–96.
23. Epstein JB, Smutzer G, Doty RL. Understanding the impact of taste changes in oncology care. *Support Care Cancer* 2016;24:1917–31.
24. Ponticelli E et al. Dysgeusia and health-related quality of life of cancer patients receiving chemotherapy: A cross-sectional study. *Eur J Cancer Care* 2017;26(2).
25. Sibaud V et al. Dermatological adverse events with taxane chemotherapy. *Eur J Dermatol* 2016;26:427–43.
26. Van der Veen J, Nuyts S. Can intensity-modulated-radiotherapy reduce toxicity in head and neck squamous cell carcinoma? *Cancer* 2017;9(10).
27. Sroussi HY et al. Common oral complications of head and neck cancer radiation therapy: Mucositis, infections, saliva change, fibrosis, sensory dysfunctions, dental caries, periodontal disease, and osteoradionecrosis. *Cancer Med* Epub October 25. 2017.
28. Maria OM, Eliopoulos N, Muanza T. Radiation-induced oral mucositis. *Front Oncol* 2017;7:89.
29. Elad S, Zadik Y. Chronic oral mucositis after radiotherapy to the head and neck: A new insight. *Support Care Cancer* 2016;24:4825–30.
30. Hartl DM et al. Otorhinolaryngological toxicities of new drugs in oncology. *Adv Ther* 2017;34:866–94.
31. de Bataille C et al. Management of radiation-induced mucosal necrosis with photobiomodulation therapy. *Support Care Cancer* Epub October 9, 2017.
32. Mercadante V et al. Interventions for the management of radiotherapy-induced xerostomia and hyposalivation: A systematic review and meta-analysis. *Oral Oncol* 2017;66:64–74.

33. Buglione M et al. Oral toxicity management in head and neck cancer patients treated with chemotherapy and radiation: Xerostomia and trismus (Part 2). Literature review and consensus statement. *Crit Rev Oncol Hematol* 2016;102:47–54.

34. Yang WF et al. Is pilocarpine effective in preventing radiation-induced xerostomia? A systematic review and meta-analysis. *Int J Radiat Oncol Biol Phys* 2016;94:503–11.

35. Sibaud V et al. Oral toxicity of targeted anticancer therapies. *Ann Dermatol Venereol* 2014;141:354–63.

36. Watters AL, Epstein JB, Agulnik M. Oral complications of targeted cancer therapies: A narrative literature review. *Oral Oncol* 2011;47:441–8.

37. Yuan A et al. Oral adverse events in cancer patients treated with VEGFR-directed multitargeted tyrosine kinase inhibitors. *Oral Oncol* 2015;51:1026–33.

38. Boers-Doets CB et al. Oral adverse events associated with tyrosine kinase and mammalian target of rapamycin inhibitors in renal cell carcinoma: A structured literature review. *Oncologist* 2012;17:135–44.

39. Peterson DE et al. Oral mucosal injury caused by mammalian target of rapamycin inhibitors: Emerging perspectives on pathobiology and impact on clinical practice. *Cancer Med* 2016;5:1897–907.

40. Jensen SB, Peterson DE. Oral mucosal injury caused by cancer therapies: Current management and new frontiers in research. *J Oral Pathol Med* 2014;43:81–90.

41. Yuan A, Woo SB. Adverse drug events in the oral cavity. *Oral Surg Oral Med Oral Path Oral Rad* 2015;119:35–47.

42. Reyes-Habito CM, Roh EK. Cutaneous reactions to chemotherapeutic drugs and targeted therapy for cancer: Part II. Targeted therapy. *J Am Acad Dermatol* 2014;71:217.e1–217.e11.

43. Sonis S et al. Preliminary characterization of oral lesions associated with inhibitors of mammalian target of rapamycin in cancer patients. *Cancer* 2010;116:210–5.

44. Martins F et al. A review of oral toxicity associated with mTOR inhibitor therapy in cancer patients. *Oral Oncol* 2013;49:293–8.

45. Gomez-Fernandez C et al. The risk of skin rash and stomatitis with the mammalian target of rapamycin inhibitor temsirolimus: A systematic review of the literature and meta-analysis. *Eur J Cancer* 2012;48:340–6.

46. Vargo CA et al. Occurrence and characterization of everolimus adverse events during first and subsequent cycles in the treatment of metastatic breast cancer. *Support Care Cancer* 2016;24:2913–8.

47. Rugo HS et al. Incidence and time course of everolimus-related adverse events in postmenopausal women with hormone receptor-positive advanced breast cancer: Insights from BOLERO-2. *Ann Oncol* 2014;25:808–15.

48. De Oliveira MA et al. Clinical presentation and management of mTOR inhibitor-associated stomatitis. *Oral Oncol* 2011;47:998–1003.

49. Rugo HS et al. Meta-analysis of stomatitis in clinical studies of everolimus: Incidence and relationship with efficacy. *Ann Oncol* 2016;27:519–25.

50. Rugo HS et al. Prevention of everolimus-related stomatitis in women with hormone receptor-positive, HER2-negative metastatic breast cancer using dexamethasone mouthwash (SWISH): A single-arm, phase 2 trial. *Lancet Oncol* 2017;18:654–62.

51. Macdonald JB, Macdonald B, Golitz LE, LoRusso P, Sekulic A. Cutaneous adverse effects of targeted therapies: Part II: Inhibitors of intracellular molecular signaling pathways. *J Am Acad Dermatol* 2015;72(2):221–36.

52. Melosky B, Hirsh V. Management of common toxicities in metastatic NSCLC related to anti-lung cancer therapies with EGFR-TKIs. *Front Oncol* 2014;4:238.

53. Elting LS et al. Risk of oral and gastrointestinal mucosal injury among patients receiving selected targeted agents: A meta-analysis. *Support Care Cancer* 2013;21:3243–54.

54. Miroddi M et al. Risk of grade 3-4 diarrhea and mucositis in colorectal cancer patients receiving anti-EGFR monoclonal antibodies regimens: A meta-analysis of 18 randomized controlled clinical trials. *Crit Rev Oncol Hematol* 2015;96:355–71.

55. Bonner JA et al. Radiotherapy plus cetuximab for squamous-cell carcinoma of the head and neck. *N Engl J Med* 2006;354:567–78.

56. Tejwani A et al. Increased risk of high-grade dermatologic toxicities with radiation plus epidermal growth factor receptor inhibitor therapy. *Cancer* 2009;115:1286–99.

57. Lacouture ME et al. Clinical practice guidelines for the prevention and treatment of EGFR inhibitor-associated dermatologic toxicities. *Support Care Cancer* 2011;19:1079–95.
58. Lacouture ME et al. A proposed EGFR inhibitor dermatologic adverse event-specific grading scale from the MASCC skin toxicity study group. *Support Care Cancer* 2010;18:509–22.
59. Kollmannsberger C et al. Sunitinib in metastatic renal cell carcinoma: Recommendations for management of non-cardiovascular toxicities. *Oncologist* 2011;16:543–53.
60. Elisei R et al. Cabozantinib in progressive medullary thyroid cancer. *J Clin Oncol* 2013;31:3639–46.
61. Ibrahim EM et al. Sunitinib adverse events in metastatic renal cell carcinoma: A meta-analysis. *Int J Clin Oncol* 2013;18:1060–9.
62. Edmonds K et al. Strategies for assessing and managing the adverse events of sorafenib and other targeted therapies in the treatment of renal cell and hepatocellular carcinoma: Recommendations from a European nursing task group. *Eur J Oncol Nurs* 2012;16:172–84.
63. Gavrilovic IT et al. Characteristics of oral mucosal events related to bevacizumab treatment. *Oncologist* 2012;17:274–8.
64. Hubiche T et al. Geographic tongue induced by angiogenesis inhibitors. *Oncologist* 2013;18:e16–17.
65. Christodoulou C et al. Combination of bisphosphonates and antiangiogenic factors induces osteonecrosis of the jaw more frequently than bisphosphonates alone. *Oncology* 2009;76:209–11.
66. Gómez Fernández C et al. Oral lichenoid eruption associated with imatinib treatment. *Eur J Dermatol* 2010;20:127–8.
67. Amitay-Laish I, Stemmer SM, Lacouture ME. Adverse cutaneous reactions secondary to tyrosine kinase inhibitors including imatinib mesylate, nilotinib, and dasatinib. *Dermatol Ther* 2011;24:386–95.
68. Basso FG et al. Skin and oral lesions associated to imatinib mesylate therapy. *Support Care Cancer* 2009;17:465–8.
69. Fitzpatrick SG, Hirsch SA, Gordon SC. The malignant transformation of oral lichen planus and oral lichenoid lesions: A systematic review. *J Am Dent Assoc* 2014;145:45–56.
70. Khoo TL et al. Hyperpigmentation of the hard palate associated with imatinib therapy for chronic myeloid leukemia with a genetic variation in the proto-oncogene c-KIT. *Leuk Lymphoma* 2013;54:186–8.
71. Balagula Y et al. Pigmentary changes in a patient treated with imatinib. *J Drugs Dermatol* 2011;10:1062–6.
72. Boussemart L et al. Prospective study of cutaneous side-effects associated with the BRAF inhibitor vemurafenib: A study of 42 patients. *Ann Oncol* 2013;24:1691–7.
73. Vigarios E et al. Oral squamous cell carcinoma and hyperkeratotic lesions with BRAF inhibitors. *Br J Dermatol* 2015;172:1680–2.
74. Mangold AR, Bryce A, Sekulic A. Vemurafenib-associated gingival hyperplasia in patient with metastatic melanoma. *J Am Acad Dermatol* 2014;71:e205–6.
75. Nogova L et al. Evaluation of BGJ398, a fibroblast growth factor receptor 1-3 kinase inhibitor, in patients with advanced solid tumors harboring genetic alterations in fibroblast growth factor receptors: Results of a global phase I, dose-escalation and dose-expansion study. *J Clin Oncol* 2017;35:157–65.
76. Tabernero J et al. Phase I dose-escalation study of JNJ-42756493, an oral pan-fibroblast growth factor receptor inhibitor, in patients with advanced solid tumors. *J Clin Oncol* 2015;33:3401–8.
77. Bétrian S et al. Severe onycholysis and eyelash trichomegaly following use of new selective pan-FGFR inhibitors. *JAMA Dermatol* 2017;153:723–5.
78. Sibaud V et al. Ado-trastuzumab emtansine-associated telangiectasias in metastatic breast cancer: A case series. *Breast Cancer Res Treat* 2014;146:423–6.
79. Sibaud V et al. T-DM1-related telangiectasias: A potential role in secondary bleeding events. *Ann Oncol* 2015;26:436–7.
80. Solomon BJ et al. First-line crizotinib versus chemotherapy in ALK-positive lung cancer. *N Engl J Med* 2014;371:2167–77.
81. Basset-Seguin N et al. Vismodegib in patients with advanced basal cell carcinoma (STEVIE): A pre-planned interim analysis of an international, open-label trial. *Lancet Oncol* 2015;16:729–36.
82. Sekulic A et al. Efficacy and safety of vismodegib in advanced basal-cell carcinoma. *N Engl J Med* 2012;366:2171–9.
83. Rizvi NA et al. Activity and safety of nivolumab, an anti-PD-1 immune checkpoint inhibitor, for patients with advanced, refractory squamous non-small-cell lung cancer (CheckMate 063): A phase 2, single-arm trial. *Lancet Oncol* 2015;16:257–65.

84. Topalian SL et al. Survival, durable tumor remission, and long-term safety in patients with advanced melanoma receiving nivolumab. *J Clin Oncol* 2014;32:1020–30.

85. McDermott DF et al. Atezolizumab, an anti-programmed death-ligand 1 antibody, in metastatic renal cell carcinoma: Long-term safety, clinical activity, and immune correlates from a phase Ia study. *J Clin Oncol* 2016;34:833–42.

86. Haanen JBAG et al. Management of toxicities from immunotherapy: ESMO Clinical Practice Guidelines for diagnosis, treatment and follow-up. *Ann Oncol* 2017;28:iv119–42.

87. Shi VJ et al. Clinical and histologic features of lichenoid mucocutaneous eruptions due to anti-programmed cell death 1 and anti-programmed cell death ligand 1 immunotherapy. *JAMA Dermatol* 2016;152:1128–36.

88. Rapoport BL et al. Supportive care for patients undergoing immunotherapy. *Support Care Cancer* Epub July 13, 2017.

89. Naidoo J et al. Toxicities of the anti-PD-1 and anti-PD-L1 immune checkpoint antibodies. *Ann Oncol* 2015;26:2375–91.

90. Hofmann L et al. Cutaneous, gastrointestinal, hepatic, endocrine, and renal side-effects of anti-PD-1 therapy. *Eur J Cancer* 2016;60:190–209.

91. Schaberg KB et al. Immunohistochemical analysis of lichenoid reactions in patients treated with anti-PD-L1 and anti-PD-1 therapy. *J Cutan Pathol* 2016;43:339–46.

92. Sibaud V et al. Oral lichenoid reactions associated with anti-PD-1/PD-L1 therapies: Clinicopathological findings. *J Eur Acad Dermatol Venereol* 2017;31:e464–9.

9

Chemotherapeutic-Induced Nail Reactions

Eric Wong, Maria Carmela Annunziata, and Antonella Tosti

Chemotherapy is a common etiology of adverse effects seen in the nails. Nail abnormalities are typically caused by acute damage, and clinical features are dependent on which component of the nail apparatus is affected (1). The nail apparatus is composed of the matrix, nail bed, nail plate, hyponychium, and proximal and lateral nail folds (2). Nail changes may develop immediately after exposure to the medication or after a few months of treatment. Recovery can be slow as the nail unit grows at a rate of 3 and 1 mm per month for the fingernails and toenails, respectively (3). Most nail abnormalities due to chemotherapy affect several or all nails (4).

Symptoms vary from no symptoms to painful and discomforting and in some cases patients need to interrupt the treatment because of the nail changes (4). Yet although some of these changes can be permanent, most often nail abnormalities are reversed once medications are withdrawn (1).

Drug-Induced Nail Matrix Damage

Medications that cause an acute decrease or arrest in mitotic activity of the keratinocytes of the nail matrix can cause a variability of signs from a mild thinning or decreased nail growth to a full cessation of nail plate growth (3). Physicians should inquire about potential medications or drugs, most commonly initiated within 2–3 weeks prior to the onset of nail symptoms. Changes that can be seen include nail thinning/brittleness, changes in the nail growth rate and arrest of nail plate production, and impaired mitotic activity of the keratinocytes.

Nail Thinning/Brittleness

Chemotherapeutic medications, such as taxanes, bruton tyrosine kinase inhibitors (including ibrutinib) and BRAF inhibitors (vemurafenib), and EGFR (epidermal growth factor receptor) inhibitors can alter production of nail plates and thus cause nail thinning and brittleness (Figure 9.1) (1,4–7). Although the pathogenesis of chemotherapy-induced brittle nails is not known, it is suggested that there is a multifactorial cause, including damage of the matrix causing alteration of nail plate production, damage to the already keratinized nail plate, or underlying poor metabolic or nutritional health in patient with advanced cancer (1,3,8).

Treatment of thin and brittle nails can include prevention of trauma and repeated water exposure via rubber gloves, routine maintenance of nail hygiene by keeping nails short, avoidance of irritants and nail polish removers (which can cause dehydration), and use of nail moisturizers (including occlusive and humectants) (9). Over time, oral supplementation with biotin (5 mg/daily) vitamin may help strengthen nails (10). Nail lacquers (hydroxypropyl chitosan and poly-ureaurethane 16%) have been approved for brittle nails by the U.S. Food and Drug Administration (8).

Changes in Nail Growth Rate

Chemotherapeutic agents, including methotrexate, have shown to decrease nail growth rate (11). Nail growth rate typically will return to normal once the drug is discontinued (3).

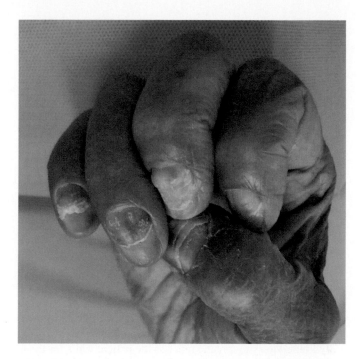

FIGURE 9.1 Onychomadesis, onycholysis, and brittle nails in a patient treated with erlotinib.

Beau's Lines/Onychomadesis

Beau's lines present as transverse depressions or indentations occurring on the nail plate (Figure 9.2) (3,12). Onychomadesis, a term to describe a more severe variant of Beau's lines, presents as a separation or shedding of the nail from the proximal nail fold (Figure 9.1) (19). The length and size of the depression can give the physician an indication regarding the duration and severity of insult of the offending source on the nail matrix (1). They typically affect most or all nails and each nail usually presents multiple lines, each corresponding to a cycle of chemotherapy.

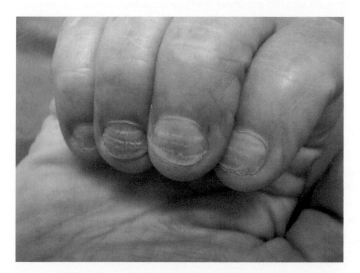

FIGURE 9.2 Beau's lines presenting as transverse depressions of the nail plate corresponding with each cycle of chemotherapy.

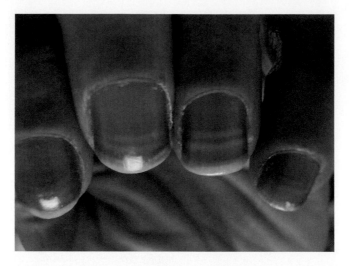

FIGURE 9.3   True leukonychia: transverse parallel white lines developing after each cycle of chemotherapy.

Chemotherapeutic agents most often associated with nail matrix damage include taxanes, cisplatin, melphalan, and vincristine (1,13–17). Beau's lines or onychomadesis resolve with nail growth (20).

Treatment is generally limited to symptomatic relief as the patient waits for the nail to grow out (11).

True Transverse Leukonychia

Medications that impair the mitotic activity of the keratinocytes located in the distal nail matrix cause parakeratosis (or retention of nuclei) of the ventral nail plate with transverse leukonychia. As opposed to apparent leukonychia (see later), true transverse leukonychia presents as opaque, persistent, white bands, typically 1–2 mm in width that move distally with nail growth (Figure 9.3). They do not resolve when pressure is applied to them (12). As for Beau's lines, nails often present multiple bands corresponding to repeated cycles of chemotherapy.

Chemotherapeutic agents that have been associated with true transverse leukonychia include daunorubicin, doxorubicin, cyclophosphamide, vincristine, and arsenic for treatment of acute myeloid leukemia (11). There is no specific treatment for transverse leukonychia, as the nail plate will grow out with time (3).

Drug-Induced Nail Pigmentation (Melanonychia)

Melanonychia is a black or brown longitudinal or transverse pigmentation of the nail plate due to production of melanin pigment from activated melanocytes in nail matrix (Figure 9.4) (1,3,18,19). Drug-induced melanonychia usually affects several or all nails and presents as soon as 3–8 weeks after starting a medication (Figure 9.5). It can be associated with other skin and mucosal pigmentation, and with other nail abnormalities due to chemotherapy (8). This discoloration can be reversible once the drug is stopped, however, this may take weeks to months to allow the nail to grow out (11). Chemotherapeutic agents most commonly reported in causing melanonychia include hydroxyurea (hydroxycarbamide), methotrexate, bleomycin, cyclophosphamide, anthracyclines (daunorubicin), and 5-fluorouracil (18,21).

Drug-Induced Nail Bed Damage

Onycholysis

Damage to nail bed causes nail plate detachment with onycholysis (Figure 9.1). Onycholysis, due to chemotherapeutic agents, is usually hemorrhagic and painful (1). In patients treated with taxanes,

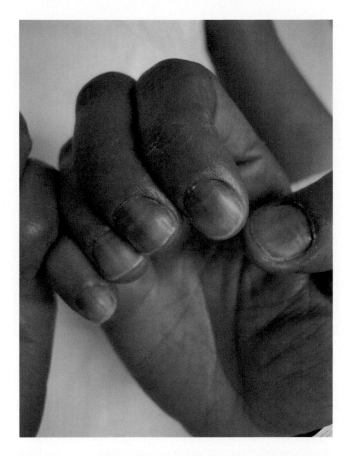

FIGURE 9.4   Muehrcke's lines (apparent leukonychia) and melanonychia in a patient undergoing polychemotherapy.

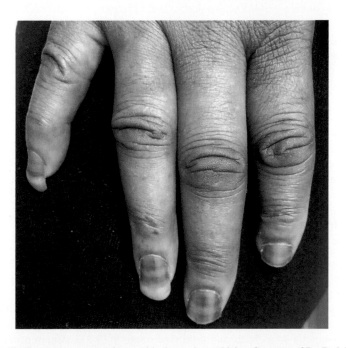

FIGURE 9.5   Longitudinal and transverse melanonychia due to doxorubicin. (Courtesy of Dr. Beth McLellan.)

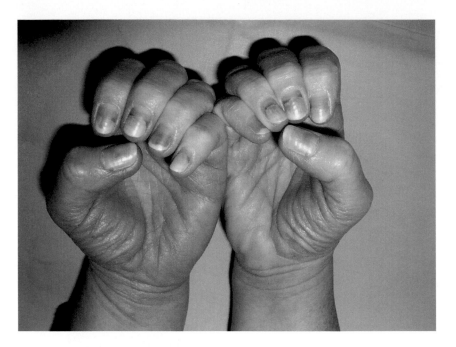

FIGURE 9.6   Hemorrhagic onycholysis in a patient on taxanes.

painful hemorrhagic onycholysis can undergo secondary bacterial infection with formation of subungual abscesses (Figure 9.6) (20). It is thought that this is from the medications' toxic effect on the nail bed disrupting angiogenesis. Pain is present due to pressure and can be relieved by manual/surgical drainage. The subungual abscesses can potentially lead to severe complications, including sepsis, especially in neutropenic patients. Chemotherapy regimens with taxanes are believed to increase susceptibility of bacterial infections due to their immunosuppressive effects (13,22–26). BRAF inhibitors (dabrafenib), capecitabine, etoposide, fluorouracil, mitoxantrone, and doxorubicin can also cause onycholysis (1,5,8,16,27–30).

Onycholysis is generally thought to be reversible once the inciting factors are discontinued. In some cases, onycholysis can resolve without stopping the medications. Therefore, treatment is generally symptomatic. Suggestions may include soaking fingers in antiseptic solution to prevent secondary microbial colonization and decrease infection rate, routine hand hygiene via clipping nonadhered nails as short as possible, gentle drying after hand washing, avoiding contact irritants, and prevention and protection of trauma with gloves (9,11).

Treatment of subungual abscesses include antibiotics and/or cyclooxygenase-2 inhibitors (31). Cryotherapy (at a temperature of −30°C) through the application of frozen gloves or socks can be considered to prevent/reduce the side effect instead of discontinuation of the medication (4,32).

Apparent Leukonychia

Apparent leukonychia present as parallel, white bands that disappear with pressure. As opposed to true leukonychia, apparent leukonychia does not migrate with growth of the nail plate (1). The exact pathogenesis of leukonychia is unknown, but they are believed to be caused by damage to the nail bed vessels leading to variable blood flow (1,18,11). Muehrcke's nails are a typical example of apparent leukonychia due to chemotherapy (Figure 9.4) (8). Apparent leukonychia is a common side effect of combined chemotherapy. It has also been in reported patients on doxorubicin and tyrosine kinase inhibitors (TKIs), including sorafebnib, sunitinib, and imatinib (8,33). Apparent leukonychia typically resolves with discontinuation of medication (18).

Drug-Induced Damage to the Proximal Nail Fold

Acute Paronychia

Paronychia presents as tender and painful inflammation of the proximal or lateral nail folds (18). Although the pathogenesis of paronychia is poorly understood, drug-induced paronychia is thought to be related with penetration of fragile nail pieces into the periungual area and typically occurs within 1–3 months of initiation of medications (11). Chemotherapeutic agents that can cause this side effect include methotrexate, MEK (mitogen-activated protein kinase) inhibitors (including selumetinib, trametinib, cobimetinib), EGFR inhibitors (such as panitumumab, gefitinib, cetuximab, and lapatinib), and BRAF inhibitors for metastatic melanoma (vemurafenib) (5,34–39). It is estimated that 10–15% of patients can develop drug-induced paronychia while on these chemotherapeutic agents, typically a month after treatment initiation (41). Paronychia is often complicated by development of pyogenic granulomas.

Paronychia tends to regress with dose reduction or discontinuation of medications, however, treatment can include proper nail hygiene and protection, antiseptic washes, and topical corticosteroids to help decrease inflammation (1,40). Other treatments include topical povidone-iodine/dimethylsufoxide solutions, chemical cautery (with silver nitrate or ferric subsulfate), tetracycline antibiotics, topical adapalene, destructive methods (electrodesiccation), or surgical removal (partial nail-plate excision) (37,38,42–45).

Pyogenic Granulomas

Pyogenic granulomas present as small, round, red, shiny nodules that have a tendency to bleed (1). Pyogenic granulomas have been described in patients on taxanes, tyrosine kinase inhibitors (Figure 9.7), MEK inhibitors, and EGFR inhibitors such as cetuximab, and typically involve the proximal and lateral nail folds of one or more nails (4,8,33,34,37,39). Typically, discontinuing medications can improve symptoms, but sometimes topical corticosteroids and/or mupirocin ointment may help improve symptoms and prevent infection (11,12). Other treatments that can be considered include topical alitretinoin (9-*cis*-retinoic acid), cauterization of the granuloma with 8% phenol solution, topical application of liquid nitrogen, topical steroids, or weekly 10% aqueous silver nitrate. Surgical excision is possible but lesions may recur (8,11,46–48). In the authors' experience, photodynamic therapy can also be a useful treatment.

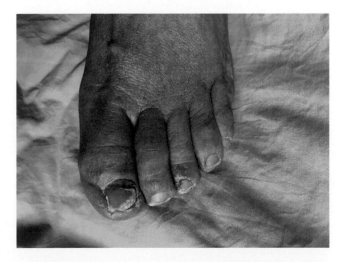

FIGURE 9.7 Paronychia and pyogenic granulomas from afatinib. (Courtesy of Dr. Beth McLellan.)

Drug-Induced Nail Blood Flow Changes

Ischemia

Ischemia occurs when perfusion to tissue is compromised, leading potentially to necrosis. Ischemia can progress from Raynaud's phenomenon to gangrene if blood circulation is not restored. Raynaud's phenomenon is the initial sign of ischemia and is a result of vasospasm of arteries causing reduced blood flow. Symptoms may be irreversible, and limb or digit amputation may be required if ischemia persists too long. Systemic or intralesional bleomycin therapy for treatment of germ cell testicular cancer has been described to cause digital and nail ischemia (11,49).

Subungual Hemorrhage

Subungual hemorrhage, presenting as splinter hemorrhages and subungual hematomas of the nail unit, are produced from damage of the nail unit caused by alterations in the nail bed blood flow. Splinter

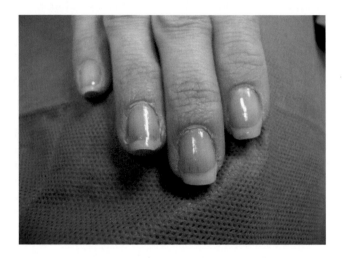

FIGURE 9.8 Splinter hemorrhages of the nail bed in a patient treated with VEGF inhibitors.

TABLE 9.1

Drug Classes and Most Common Side Effects (in Order of Most Common to Less Common)

Drug Class	Nail Abnormality	Reference
EGFR inhibitors	Paronychia with pyogenic granuloma	8, 36, 38, 47, 52
	Brittle nails	45
VEGFR inhibitors	Splinter hemorrhages	8, 33, 45
	Muehrcke's lines	33
TKIs	Paronychia	36
	Subungual splinter hemorrhages	45
MEK inhibitors	Paronychia	37
	Onycholysis	5
BRAF inhibitors	Paronychia	5
	Onycholysis	
	Brittle nails	
Taxanes	Hemorrhagic onycholysis with subungual abscesses	4, 13, 23, 26
	Onychomadesis/Beau's lines	50
	Paronychia	
	Onychorrhexis	

hemorrhages are thought to be caused by selective VEGF blocking resulting in small clots of blood vessels running vertically in the nail bed as well as thrombocytopenia. They present as short, violaceous to brown lines (Figure 9.8) (1,19). Splinter hemorrhages are typically asymptomatic and estimated to occur in 30–70% of patients, 2–4 weeks after initiation of therapy on VEGF/VEGFR. These symptoms may be suggestive of a medication effectiveness (53). Subungual hematomas are trapped red to brown blood between the nail plate and nail bed. Both lesions tend to resolve with time (11). Subungual hemorrhages and hematomas can occur with taxanes, mitoxantrone, and VEGFR, including sorafenib, sunitinib, and imatinib (26,33,45,51).

Table 9.1 summarizes the most common nail side effects by class of drug.

REFERENCES

1. Piraccini BM et al. Drug- induced nail diseases. *Dermatol Clin* 2006;24(3):387–91.
2. Haneke E. Surgical anatomy of the nail apparatus. *Dermatol Clin* 2006;24:291–6.
3. Piraccini BM, Tosti A. Drug-induced nail disorders: Incidence, management and prognosis. *Drug Saf* 1999;21(3):187–201.
4. Gilbar P, Hain A, Peereboom VM. Nail toxicity induced by cancer chemotherapy. *J Oncol Pharm Pract* 2009;15(3):143–55.
5. Dika E et al. Hair and nail adverse events during treatment with targeted therapies for metastatic melanoma. *Eur J Dermatol* 2016;26(3):232–9.
6. Bitar C et al. Hair and nail changes during long-term therapy with ibrutinib for chronic lymphocytic leukemia. *JAMA Dermatol* 2016;152(6):698–701.
7. Garden BC, Wu S, Lacouture ME. The risk of nail changes with epidermal growth factor receptor inhibitors: A systematic review of the literature and meta-analysis. *J Am Acad Dermatol* 2012;67(3):400–8.
8. Robert C et al. Nail toxicities induced by systemic anticancer treatments. *Lancet Oncol* 2015;16(4):e181–9.
9. Piraccini BM et al. Treatment of nail disorders. *Therapy* 2004;1(1):159–67.
10. Colombo VE et al. Treatment of brittle fingernails and onychoschizia with biotin: Scanning electron microscopy. *J Am Acad Dermatol* 1990;23(6 Pt 1):1127–32.
11. Piraccini BM, Iorizzo M. Drug reactions affecting the nail unit: Diagnosis and management. *Dermatol Clin* 2007;25(2):215–21, vii.
12. Piraccini BM et al. Drug- induced nail abnormalities. *Expert Opin Drug Saf* 2004;3(1):57–65.
13. Minisini AM et al. Taxane-induced nail changes: Incidence, clinical presentation and outcome. *Ann Oncol* 2003;14(2):333–7.
14. Eastwood JB et al. Shedding of nails apparently induced by the administration of large amounts of cephaloridine and cloxacillin in two anephric patients. *Br J Dermatol* 1969;81(10):750–2.
15. Chen HH, Liao YH. Beau's lines associated with itraconazole. *Acta Dermato-Venereologica* 2002;82(5):398.
16. Susser WS, Whitaker-Worth DL, Grant-Kels JM. Mucocutaneous reactions to chemotherapy. *J Am Acad Dermatol* 1999;40:367–98.
17. Vassallo C et al. Nail changes secondary to hematologic conditions. *Haematologica* 2001;86:334–6.
18. Hinds G, Thomas VD. Malignancy and cancer treatment-related hair and nail changes. *Dermatol Clin* 2008;26(1):59–68, viii.
19. Piraccini BM, Iorizzo M, Tosti A. Drug-induced nail abnormalities. *Am J Clin Dermatol* 2003;4:31–7.
20. Roh MR, Cho JY, Lew W. Docetaxel-induced onycholysis: The role of subungual hemorrhage and suppuration. *Yonsei Med J* 2007;48(1):124–6.
21. Oh ST et al. Hydroxyurea-induced melanonychia concomitant with a dermatomyositis-like eruption. *J Am Acad Dermatol* 2003;49(2):339–41.
22. Vanhooteghem O et al. Subungual abscess: A new ungula side-effect related to docetaxel therapy. *Br J Dermatol* 2000;143(2):462–4.
23. Pavithran K, Doval DC. Nail changes due to docetaxel. *Br J Dermatol* 2002;146(4):709–10.
24. Nicolopoulos J, Howard A. Docetaxel-induced nail dystrophy. *Australas J Dermatol* 2002;43(3):293–6.
25. Correia O et al. Nail changes secondary to docetaxel (Taxotere). *Dermatology* 1999;198(3):288–90.
26. Ghetti E, Piraccini BM, Tosti A. Onycholysis and subungual haemorrhages secondary to systemic chemotherapy (paclitaxel). *J Eur Acad Dermatol Venereol* 2003;17(4):459–60.

27. Chen GY et al. Onychomadesis and onycholysis associated with capecitabine. *Br J Dermatol* 2001;145:520–1.
28. Maino KL, Norwood C, Stashower ME. Onycholysis with the appearance of a "sunset" secondary to capecitabine. *Cutis* 2003;72:234–6.
29. Munoz A et al. Onycholysis associated with capecitabine in combination with irinotecan in two patients with colorectal cancer. *J Natl Cancer Inst* 2003;16:1252–3.
30. Obermair A et al. Onycholysis of the finger and toenails following the application of high-dose oral etoposide (1250 mg/m^2) given as 200 and 150 mg single doses from days 1–10 every 3 weeks. *Gynecol Oncol* 1995;57:436.
31. Nakamura S et al. Improvement in docetaxel-induced nail changes associated with cyclooxygenase-2 inhibitor treatment. *Clin Exp Dermatol* 2009;34(7):e320–1.
32. Scotté F et al. Multicenter study of a frozen glove to prevent docetaxel-induced onycholysis and cutaneous toxicity of the hand. *J Clin Oncol* 2005;23:4424–9.
33. Heidary N, Naik H, Burgin S. Chemotherapeutic agents and the skin: An update. *J Am Acad Dermatol* 2008;58(4):545–70.
34. Busam KJ et al. Cutaneous side-effects in cancer patients treated with the antiepidermal growth factor receptor antibody C225. *Br J Dermatol* 2001;144(6):1169–76.
35. Chang GC et al. Paronychia and skin hyperpigmentation induced by gefitinib in advanced non-small cell lung cancer. *J Clin Oncol* 2004;22:4646–7.
36. Lacouture ME et al. Analysis of dermatologic events in patients with cancer treated with lapatinib. *Breast Cancer Res Treat* 2009;114(3):485–93.
37. Balagula Y et al. Dermatologic side effects associated with the MEK 1/2 inhibitor, selumetinib. *Invest New Drugs* 2011;29(5):1114–21.
38. Wu PA et al. Prophylaxis and treatment of dermatologic adverse events from epidermal growth factor receptor inhibitors. *Curr Opin Oncol* 2011;23(4):343–51.
39. Schad K et al. Mitogen-activated protein/extracellular signal-regulated kinase kinase inhibition results in biphasic alteration of epidermal homeostasis with keratinocytic apoptosis and pigmentation disorders. *Clin Cancer Res* 2010;16:1058–64.
40. Piraccini BM, Iorizzo M, Tosti A. Drug-induced nail abnormalities. *Am J Clin Dermatol* 2003;4(1):31–37.
41. Deslandres M et al. Cutaneous side effects associated with epidermal growth factor receptor and tyrosine kinase inhibitors. *Ann Dermatol Venereol* 2008;1:16–24.
42. Galimont-Collen AF et al. Classification and management of skin, hair, nail and mucosal side-effects of epidermal growth factor receptor (EGFR) inhibitors. *Eur J Cancer* 2007;43(5):845–51.
43. Capriotti K et al. Chemotherapy-associated paronychia treated with 2% povidone-iodine: A series of cases. *Cancer Manag Res* 2017;9:225.
44. Hachisuka J et al. Effect of adapalene on cetuximab-induced painful periungual inflammation. *J Am Acad Dermatol* 2011;64(2):e20–1.
45. Lacouture ME, Boerner SA, Lorusso PM. Non-rash skin toxicities associated with novel targeted therapies. *Clin Lung Cancer* 2006;Suppl 1:S36–42.
46. Robert C et al. Cutaneous side-effects of kinase inhibitors and blocking antibodies. *Lancet Oncol* 2005;6:491–500.
47. Fox LP. Nail toxicity associated with epidermal growth factor receptor inhibitor therapy. *J Am Acad Dermatol* 2007;56:460–5.
48. Kiyohara Y, Yamazaki N, Kishi A. Erlotinib-related skin toxicities: Treatment strategies in patients with metastatic non-small cell lung cancer. *J Am Acad Dermatol* 2013;60:463–72.
49. Vogelzang NJ et al. Raynaud's phenomenon: A common toxicity after combination chemotherapy for testicular cancer. *Ann Intern Med* 1981;95:288–92.
50. Sibaud V et al. Dermatological adverse events with taxane chemotherapy. *Eur J Dermatol* 2016;26(5):427–43.
51. Freiman A, Bouganim N, O'Brien EA. Mitozantrone-induced onycholysis associated with subungual abscesses, paronychia, and pyogenic granuloma. *J Drugs Dermatol* 2005;4:490–1.
52. Roé E et al. Description and management of cutaneous side effects during cetuximab or erlotinib treatments: A prospective study of 30 patients. *J Am Acad Dermatol* 2006;55(3):429–37.
53. Robert C et al. Subungual splinter hemorrhages: A clinical window to inhibition of vascular endothelial growth factor receptors? *Ann Intern Med* 2005;143(4):313–4.

10

Neoplastic Reactions

Peter Arne Gerber

Background

The main strategies to treat cancer include surgery, radiotherapy, pharmacotherapy, or combinations thereof. It may seem like a paradox, but in particular radiotherapy and also certain anticancer-drugs may induce the development of neoplasms themselves. Latency until the development of neoplastic reactions may be short and reactions may occur directly associated to or even under the causative treatment. Yet neoplastic reactions may also develop years after cancer cure and cause problems in long-term cancer survivors. Of note, throughout all organ systems these subsequent neoplasms (SNs) are regarded as one of the most serious complications, and subsequent malignant neoplasms (SMNs) show the strongest association with mortality in long-term cancer survivors (1,2).

Regarding neoplastic reactions of the skin, subsequent malignant and in situ neoplasms in long-term cancer survivors are almost exclusively associated with radiotherapy (3). Yet, conventional cytotoxic chemotherapy, and in particular selected targeted cancer drugs, may cause a broad spectrum of benign and malignant neoplastic reactions. Simplified, conventional chemotherapy, on the one hand, unselectively targets all rapidly proliferating cells and tissues of the body. This includes cancer cells but also healthy cells of the hematopoietic system, the mucosa, or the hair follicle. Accordingly, side effects range from anemia and hair loss, to mucosal erosions, emesis, and others (Figure 10.1). With regard to neoplastic skin reactions, conventional chemotherapy has been associated with eruptive melanocytic macules/nevi (4,5), inflammation of actinic keratoses (6,7), and pyogenic granuloma (8).

Targeted drugs, on the other hand, have revolutionized modern cancer therapy in the last decade. Their development was and is fueled by the rapid advances in molecular biology and medicine. In fact, the identification of tumor-specific cellular and molecular characteristics has provided the opportunity to design agents that are directed against these targets. Ideally, these targeted drugs would be superior to conventional chemotherapeutics due to a higher, tumor-directed efficacy and lower undirected cytotoxic side effects. Yet, targeted therapies may also be accompanied by a broad spectrum of characteristic toxicities. These are distinct from side effects of conventional chemotherapy and are in general often better tolerated. Nevertheless, also comparably severe and wearing toxicities may occur. Since many identified tumor targets are also present in the skin, cutaneous toxicities represent some of the most frequent adverse effects of targeted anticancer drugs (9–11). Neoplastic skin reactions of targeted therapies include pyogenic granuloma (12), squamoproliferative lesions (SCPLs), and nonmelanoma skin cancer (NMSC) (13–17), as well as eruptive melanocytic macules/nevi (10,18,19).

Nonmelanoma Skin Cancer and Squamoproliferative Lesions

A nonmelanoma skin cancer (NMSC) of particular importance in cancer patients receiving BRAF-targeted therapies is the keratoacanthoma (KA). KAs develop as solitary, sometimes multiple, exophytic, dome-shaped tumors with a central ulceration that are characterized by a rapid growth over few weeks (Figure 10.2). The tumor is regarded as low grade and proposed to heal without therapy under the extrusion of a central mass of debris. The occurrence of multiple NMSCs in a field of actinic skin damage

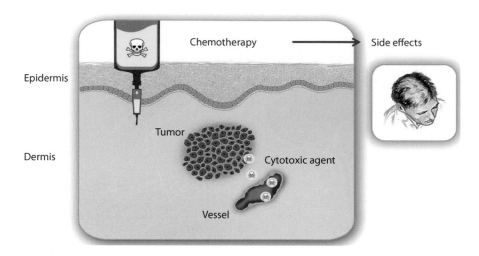

FIGURE 10.1   Conventional cytotoxic chemotherapy targets rapidly proliferating cells and tissues, for example, cancer tissue. Since this effect is relatively unselective, physiologic tissue with high proliferation rates, for example, hair follicles or mucosa, are affected. The consequences are classic chemotherapy-associated side effects such as hair loss. (Images designed by Peter Arne Gerber and Holger Schrumpf.)

is a common clinical finding and is also referred to as "actinic field cancerization" (Figure 10.3) (20). In survivors of childhood cancer, a history of radiotherapy was correlated to the development of NMSC, mainly actinic keratoses (AKs) and squamous cell carcinomas (SCCs), in 90% of affected patients (3). Yet surprisingly, no association has been identified for a positive history of conventional chemotherapy, despite its potential immunomodulating effects (please also refer to section "Neoplastic Skin Reactions in Cancer Survivors") (3). An increased risk for the development of NMSC, however, has been reported for antimetabolite hydroxyurea (HU) with latency periods of 2–13 years (21). These include multiple aggressive SCCs, Bowen's disease, and AKs in sun-exposed areas. Discontinuation of HU is proposed to result in a resolution or at least improvement of respective HU-associated squamous dysplasias. The proposed mode of action is that HU induces p53-initiated mutant keratinocytes in UV-exposed areas (21). Conventional chemotherapy has been mainly associated with reactions of preexisting NMSC, such as an induction of inflammation of AKs by 5-fluorouracil (5-FU). Pathogenetic concepts propose an increased susceptibility of transformed keratinocytes toward 5-FU–induced cell injury, resulting in subsequent inflammatory reactions (6,7).

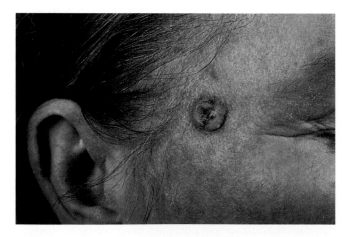

FIGURE 10.2   Keratoacanthoma.

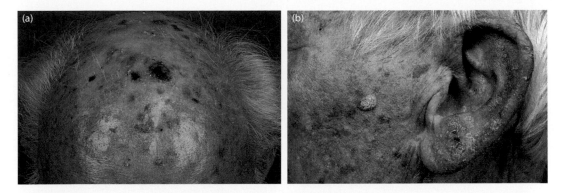

FIGURE 10.3 Clinical spectrum of nonmelanoma skin cancer (NMSC). (a) Actinic field cancerization of the scalp with multiple actinic keratoses. (b) Actinic field cancerization of the face and ear with multiple actinic and seborrheic keratoses, lentigines solares, and a verruca vulgaris.

Regarding NMSC and targeted cancer therapies, inhibitors of certain kinases of the mitogen-activated protein kinase pathway (MAPK; Figure 10.4) have been associated to a frequent induction of NMSC (AK, SCC, KA) and NMSC-like so-called keratotic or SCPLs (22). A prominent example for the importance of MAPK-signaling for the pathogenesis of solid cancer is melanoma (23). Activating mutations of the kinase BRAF are very frequent and occur in 40–60% of cutaneous melanomas (Figure 10.5). Recently, specific BRAF inhibitors, such as vemurafenib or dabrafenib, have been shown to improve both progression-free and overall survival of patients with metastatic melanoma (24,25). The application of BRAF inhibitors is associated with a spectrum of characteristic cutaneous side effects, including secondary skin tumors. The development of SCPLs, including verrucous papillomas, seborrheic keratoses, verrucae vulgares, KAs and AKs up to well-differentiated cutaneous SCCs, can be regarded as class-specific and has been reported in

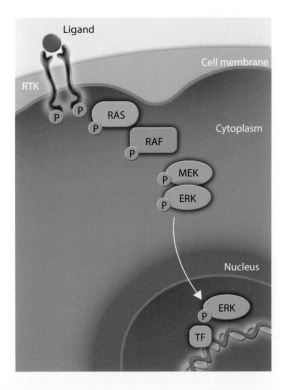

FIGURE 10.4 The EGFR/MAPK signaling pathway. (Images designed by Peter Arne Gerber and Holger Schrumpf.)

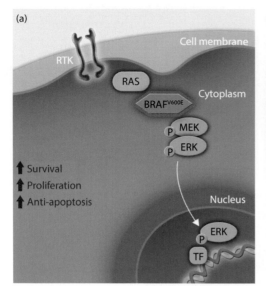
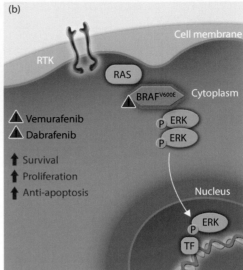
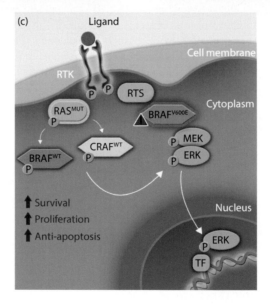

FIGURE 10.5 Altered MAPK signaling in malignant melanoma. (a) Activating BRAF-mutations (e.g., V600E) are crucial events in melanoma pathogenesis. (b) BRAF inhibitors (vemurafenib, dabrafenib) have significantly advanced modern melanoma therapy. (c) Paradoxical activation of RAS signaling is the crucial event in the pathogenesis of BRAF inhibitor–induced squamous cell proliferative lesions (SCPLs). (Images designed by Peter Arne Gerber and Holger Schrumpf.)

10–30% of the patients (Figure 10.6) (22,24,26–28). First SCPLs may appear as early as 2 weeks and up to 14 weeks after initiation of BRAF-inhibitor therapy. Molecular analyses of BRAF inhibitor–induced SCPLs have detected high frequencies of mutated RAS, particularly HRAS (27,29). Moreover, it was demonstrated that activated RAS results in a paradoxical activation of MAPK signaling and consecutive tumor growth in BRAF wild-type skin cells (27). Since these cutaneous alterations also show an overlap with a group of genetic syndromes with activating RAS/MAPK germline mutations, such as Costello or Noonan syndrome, skin side effects are also referred to as "RASopathic" (30). Concerning additional risk factors for the induction of SCPLs by RAF inhibitors, the DNA of human papillomavirus (HPV) was identified in SCPLs of patients treated with vemurafenib. Moreover, vemurafenib treatment significantly increased SCC incidence from 22 to 70% in a transgenic mouse model of HPV-driven SCC (31).

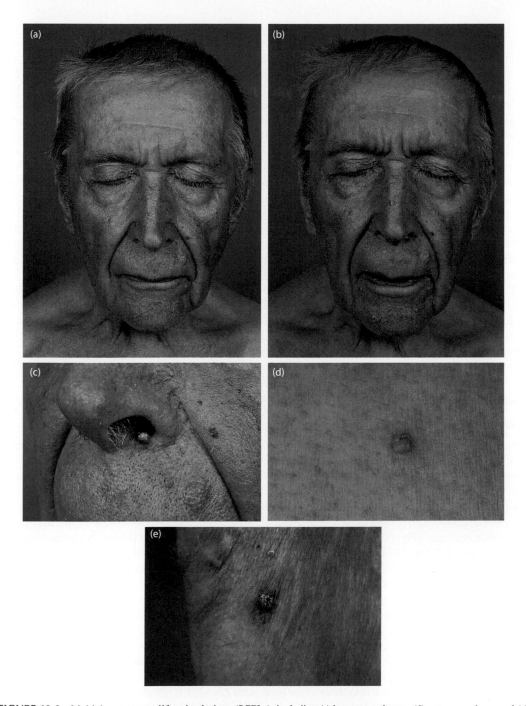

FIGURE 10.6 Multiple squamoproliferative lesions (SCPLs), including (c) keratoacanthoma, (d) cutaneous horn and (e) verrucous papilloma, in a patient treated with the BRAF inhibitor vemurafenib. Patient at (a) week 3 and (b–e) week 8 after start of BRAF inhibition.

Recommendations for the management and prevention of SCPLs in patients treated with RAF inhibitors include regular skin monitorings every 4–6 weeks and strict sun precautions. With regard to therapy of RAF inhibitor–induced neoplastic reactions, a complete surgical excision of suspect lesions is recommended (32). Yet, patients presenting with multiple lesions can also be treated with directed destructive measures, such as cryotherapy, as well as established therapies for the management of actinic field cancerization, such as topical 5-FU, ingenol mebutate, or photodynamic therapy (PDT), or combinations thereof, such as Lesion intensified field therapy (LIFT)–PDT (22,33). Finally, successful treatments have been demonstrated for oral acitretin (28). Regarding the efficacy of acitretin, it is proposed that retinoids directly interact with components of RAF/MEK/ERK and PTEN/PI13/AKT/mTOR pathways and reduce both Erk1 activity and secretion of EGF (34).

Of note, due to the advances in melanoma therapy, the induction of neoplastic reactions in patients treated with BRAF inhibitors has regressed to a negligible problem. In fact, in patients with BRAF-positive advanced melanoma, monotherapy with BRAF inhibitors have been replaced by combinations of BRAF inhibitors (vemurafenib, dabrafenib) and MEK inhibitors (trametinib, cobimetinib) as a new standard of care (35). Surprisingly, whereas the inhibition of two consecutive kinases of the MAPK pathway has significantly increased efficacy and patient's overall survival as compared to respective monotherapies, we also observed a strikingly reduced frequency of adverse effects (36). In particular, the incidence of SCPLs was reduced from 10 to 30% in BRAF inhibitor–treated to 0–1% in BRAF/MEK inhibitor–treated patients (22,35). The proposed molecular mechanism is the inhibition of paradoxical RAS signaling on the level of MEK. Strikingly, in a "proof-of-concept" observation, the addition of a MEK inhibitor to the BRAF inhibitor regime was also reported to result in the complete regression of preexisting BRAF inhibitor–induced SCPLs (37).

The induction of NMSC, including SCCs, is also associated with multikinase inhibitors (MKIs) that target RAF, such as sorafenib. Moreover, inflammatory reactions of preexisting AKs have been observed in 10% of patients treated with sorafenib (13–17,22). Finally, recent observations report the induction of KAs and SCCs in patients treated with a monoclonal antibody directed against transforming growth factor beta (anti-TGFβ), fresolimumab. In line with findings for the induction of SCPLs by RAF inhibitors, the authors propose that a crosstalk of TGFβ- and MAPK pathways is the most probable causative molecular mechanism (38).

Pigmented Lesions

Eruptive nevi associated with medications (ENAMs) have been described for a broad spectrum of pharmacologic agents, including conventional chemotherapy and targeted anticancer drugs (5). The diagnosis of ENAM can be defined by the development of >5 melanocytic nevi on palmae or plantae at any age, >10 melanocytic nevi bodywide outside of puberty or pregnancy, or (3) >10 melanocytic nevi bodywide outside of puberty or pregnancy during a period of 6 months associated with medication use (5). Nevi develop within weeks to months of therapy and often present as light- to dark-brown macules of 1–3 mm in diameter (Figure 10.7). Drug-induced nevi often present in one of the following distributions: palmoplantar; localized to the trunk; or diffuse, with a strong predilection for palms and soles (39). ENAMs can be further classified into subtypes according to the type of medication, namely, Ia "non-biologic immunosuppressants," Ib "biologic immunosuppressants," IIa "non-biologic chemotherapeutics," IIb "biologic chemotherapeutics," and III "direct melanocyte stimulators" (5).

Conventional chemotherapeutics that have been associated with ENAMs (type IIa) are capecitabine (40), interferon α-2b (41), cyclophosphamide, octreotide, doxorubicin and daunorubicin (4,6), and combination chemotherapies (5,42). Pathogenetic concepts for the induction of ENAMs by nonbiologic drugs mainly propose immunosuppressive effects and a consecutive modulation of local growth factors, such as stem cell factor (SCF) and melanocyte growth factors (39,43).

Targeted cancer drugs that have been associated with ENAMs (type IIb) include EGFR inhibitors (erlotinib) (44), BRAF inhibitors (vemurafenib, encorafenib) (45,46), and multikinase inhibitors (MKI; sorafenib, sunitinib, regorafenib) (18,19,47), as well as anti-CD20 antibodies (rituximab) (5). For BRAF inhibitors ENAMs have been reported to occur in 10% of treated patients (45). Of note, also the development of second primary melanomas (SPMs) has been described in 20% of patients treated with BRAF inhibitors (48). In line with pathogenic concepts for the induction of SCPLs and NMSCs by BRAF inhibitors and MKIs, the induction of ENAMs and SPMs by targeted drugs is the paradoxical activation of RAS-RAF-MEK signaling pathways. Again, proof-of-concept observations report the rapid and complete regression of BRAF inhibitor–induced ENAMs after escalation to a combined BRAF/MEK-inhibitor regime (45).

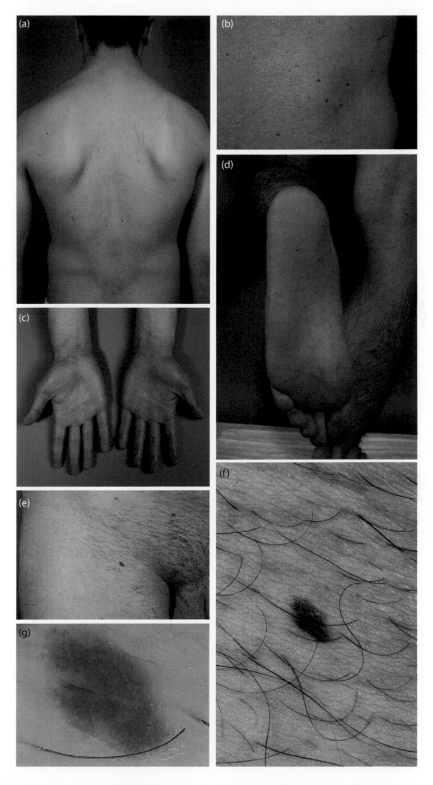

FIGURE 10.7 Eruptive nevi associated with medication (ENAM). (a–d) Back, abdomen, palms, sole. (e–g) Melanocytic nevus; overview, detail, and dermatoscopic image.

Recommendations for prevention and management of ENAMs and SPMs in patients undergoing monotherapy with BRAF inhibitors include the documentation of preexisting melanocytic nevi prior to therapy initiation ("body mapping"), monitoring visits every 4–8 weeks, including dermatoscopy and digital tracking if available, as well as strict sun precautions (22).

Pyogenic Granuloma

Pyogenic granuloma (Figure 10.8) has been associated with conventional chemotherapies such as 5-FU, capecitabine, methotrexate, and doxorubicin, as well with targeted therapies directed against EGFR (Figure 10.9), BRAF, and CD20 (12,49–52). The tumor frequently arises in periungual locations. Whereas these clinical observations link the induction of pyogenic granuloma with an inhibition of the EGFR/MAPK pathway, recent studies have identified activating RAF and RAS mutations as major drivers in the pathogenesis of pyogenic granuloma (53). These seemingly controversial findings illustrate the complex interplay of different signaling routes and kinases in the pathogenesis of targeted drugs. In line with pathogenetic models for the development of other neoplasia under EGFR/MAPK-targeting drugs, the development of pyogenic granuloma under EGFR and BRAF inhibition has contributed to a paradoxical activation of the MAPK pathway (52,54). Yet, it seems likely that pyogenic granuloma may just be the consequence of minor trauma and the increased frequency of additional toxicities of the nails and periungual area in patients treated with anticancer drugs.

Strategies for the prevention of periungual lesions and nail toxicities in patients receiving pharmacologic anticancer therapies include the avoidance of trauma or manipulations of the nails and periungual tissue as well as consequent moisturizing skin care (12,50,55). In particular, manicures and pedicures, nail biting, and removal of the nail cuticle should be avoided or carried out with caution. Additional recommendations include the use of protective gloves, cotton socks, and wide-fitting footwear; regular, straight, not too short trimming, and smoothing of the nails; visiting a medical podiatrist if necessary; and avoidance of toxic reagents and detergents (50).

Recommendations for the management of pyogenic granuloma include mainly destructive measures such as cryotherapy with the application of liquid nitrogen, as well as the topical application of 10% aqueous silver nitrate, 88% phenol, or 35% trichloroacetic acid (TCA). In addition, the application of topical steroids of high potency or intralesional injection of triamcinolone suspensions can be performed. Additional intralesional treatment options that are reported in the literature are injections of ethanolamine, sodium tetradecyl sulfate, or polidocanol (49). Yet, these measures are associated with a relevant risk of necrosis of the surrounding tissue and are therefore only listed here for the sake of completeness. More invasive options include the removal by surgical curettage, electrodesiccation, or excision, as well as laser therapy with ablative CO_2 or nonablative pulsed dye lasers (PDL) (50). In severe cases, dose adjustment or even cessation and a switch of the causative anticancer drug may be necessary (50).

Neoplastic Skin Reactions in Cancer Survivors

NMSC is the most common SN in long-term cancer survivors accounting for more than 40% of all confirmed SNs (1,3). Moreover, cancer survivors that develop NMSC have a high risk to develop a second NMSC within 10 years of the first NMSC (1). Surprisingly, whereas the development of NMSC has been associated with a history of radiotherapy in 90% and whereas 90% of these NMSCs occur in the radiotherapy field, no significant association has been identified for a positive history of chemotherapy (3). Concerning anthracycline exposure even a slightly decreased risk for NMSC has been reported (3). In adults, the antimetabolite hydroxyurea (HU) has been associated to the development of multiple NMSCs. Discontinuation of HU is proposed to result in a resolution or at least improvement of respective tumors (21).

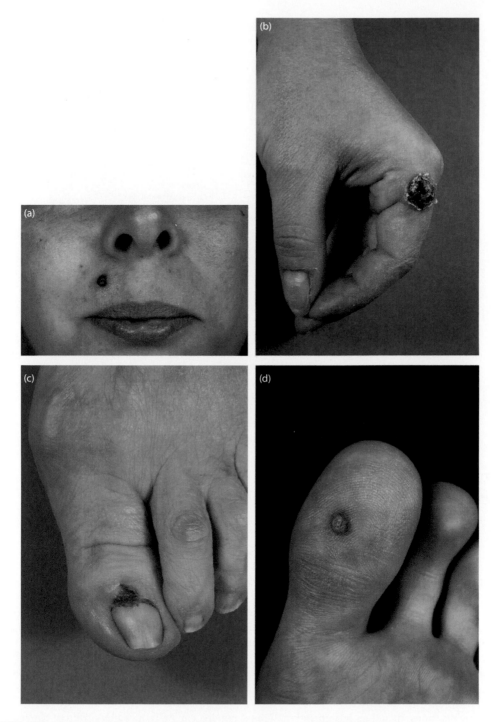

FIGURE 10.8 Pyogenic granuloma (lobular capillary hemangioma). (a–d) Clinical spectrum.

Besides NMSC, cancer survivors are also at a higher risk to develop melanoma (56,57). With regard to risk factors, chemotherapy (alkylating agents and antimitotic drugs) was only found to increase the risk of developing melanoma as an SMN in combination with radiotherapy (56). This is surprising, taking into account that chemotherapy in childhood is a well-known risk factor for the development of excess benign nevi (58). Finally, the purine analog fludarabine was recently identified to significantly increase

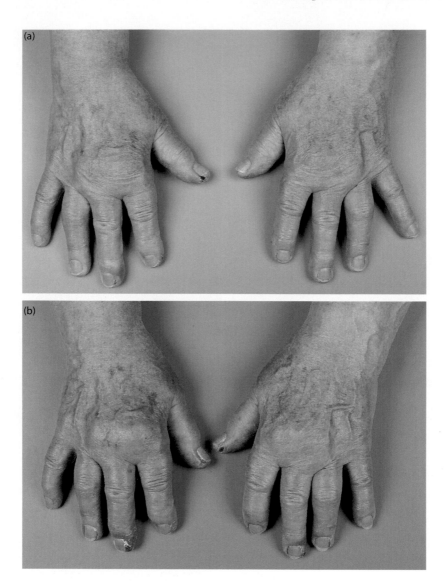

FIGURE 10.9   Skin and nail toxicities in a patient treated with the anti-EGFR antibody panitumumab: Pyogenic granuloma, paronychia and fissures. Images were taken at (a) week 6 and (b) week 8 after start of anti-EGFR treatment.

melanoma risk in survivors of chronic lymphocytic leukemia/small lymphocytic lymphoma (CLL/SLL) but not of other subtypes of non-Hodgkin lymphoma (NHL) (59).

Conclusion

Neoplastic reactions, including benign and malignant tumors, can be induced by different conventional chemotherapeutics and in particular by targeted cancer drugs. The treating oncologist should be aware of the potential spectrum and clinical presentation of respective neoplasms, as well as the recommended management options. Taking into account the dynamic developments in the field of targeted therapies and the continually growing number of novel approved drugs directed against a growing number of different targets, it is likely that the spectrum of associated neoplastic reactions also will grow. Whereas it is challenging to keep up with these advances in the field, these new reactions also offer a chance to improve our understanding of skin biology in general and of the pathogenesis of epithelial tumors in particular.

REFERENCES

1. Armstrong GT et al. Occurrence of multiple subsequent neoplasms in long-term survivors of childhood cancer: A report from the childhood cancer survivor study. *J Clin Oncol* 2011;29(22):3056–64.
2. Armstrong GT et al. Late mortality among 5-year survivors of childhood cancer: A summary from the Childhood Cancer Survivor Study. *J Clin Oncol* 2009;27(14):2328–38.
3. Perkins JL et al. Nonmelanoma skin cancer in survivors of childhood and adolescent cancer: A report from the childhood cancer survivor study. *J Clin Oncol* 2005;23(16):3733–41.
4. Lotem M et al. Skin toxic effects of polyethylene glycol-coated liposomal doxorubicin. *Arch Dermatol* 2000;136(12):1475–80.
5. Perry BM, Nguyen A, Desmond BL, Blattner CM, Thomas RS, Young RJ. Eruptive nevi associated with medications (ENAMs). *J Am Acad Dermatol* 2016;75(5):1045–52.
6. Reyes-Habito CM, Roh EK. Cutaneous reactions to chemotherapeutic drugs and targeted therapies for cancer: Part I. Conventional chemotherapeutic drugs. *J Am Acad Dermatol* 2014;71(2):203.e1–203.e12; quiz 215–16.
7. Krathen M, Treat J, James WD. Capecitabine induced inflammation of actinic keratoses. *Dermatol Online J* 2007;13(4):13.
8. Piguet V, Borradori L. Pyogenic granuloma-like lesions during capecitabine therapy. *Br J Dermatol* 2002;147(6):1270–2.
9. Agha R, Kinahan K, Bennett CL, Lacouture ME. Dermatologic challenges in cancer patients and survivors. *Oncology* 2007;21(12):1462–72; discussion 1473, 1476, 1481 passim.
10. Macdonald JB, Macdonald B, Golitz LE, LoRusso P, Sekulic A. Cutaneous adverse effects of targeted therapies: Part I: Inhibitors of the cellular membrane. *J Am Acad Dermatol* 2015;72(2):203–18; quiz 219–20.
11. Macdonald JB, Macdonald B, Golitz LE, LoRusso P, Sekulic A. Cutaneous adverse effects of targeted therapies: Part II: Inhibitors of intracellular molecular signaling pathways. *J Am Acad Dermatol* 2015;72(2):221–36; quiz 237–38.
12. Below J, Homey B, Gerber PA. [Cutaneous side effects of targeted cancer drugs]. *Hautarzt.* 2017;68(1):12–18.
13. Arnault JP et al. Keratoacanthomas and squamous cell carcinomas in patients receiving sorafenib. *J Clin Oncol* 2009;27(23):e59–61.
14. Dubauskas Z, Kunishige J, Prieto VG, Jonasch E, Hwu P, Tannir NM. Cutaneous squamous cell carcinoma and inflammation of actinic keratoses associated with sorafenib. *Clin Genitourin Cancer* 2009;7(1):20–23.
15. Kong HH, Cowen EW, Azad NS, Dahut W, Gutierrez M, Turner ML. Keratoacanthomas associated with sorafenib therapy. *J Am Acad Dermatol* 2007;56(1):171–2.
16. Lynch MC, Straub R, Adams DR. Eruptive squamous cell carcinomas with keratoacanthoma-like features in a patient treated with sorafenib. *J Drugs Dermatol* 2011;10(3):308–10.
17. Smith KJ, Haley H, Hamza S, Skelton HG. Eruptive keratoacanthoma-type squamous cell carcinomas in patients taking sorafenib for the treatment of solid tumors. *Dermatol Surg* 2009;35(11):1766–70.
18. Jimenez-Gallo D, Albarran-Planelles C, Linares-Barrios M, Martinez-Rodriguez A, Baez-Perea JM. Eruptive melanocytic nevi in a patient undergoing treatment with sunitinib. *JAMA Dermatol* 2013;149(5):624–6.
19. Kong HH, Sibaud V, Chanco Turner ML, Fojo T, Hornyak TJ, Chevreau C. Sorafenib-induced eruptive melanocytic lesions. *Arch Dermatol* 2008;144(6):820–2.
20. Stockfleth E. The paradigm shift in treating actinic keratosis: A comprehensive strategy. *J Drugs Dermatol* 2012;11(12):1462–7.
21. Sanchez-Palacios C, Guitart J. Hydroxyurea-associated squamous dysplasia. *J Am Acad Dermatol* 2004;51(2):293–300.
22. Reyes-Habito CM, Roh EK. Cutaneous reactions to chemotherapeutic drugs and targeted therapy for cancer: Part II. Targeted therapy. *J Am Acad Dermatol* 2014;71(2):217.e1–217.e11; quiz 227–28.
23. Curtin JA et al. Distinct sets of genetic alterations in melanoma. *N Engl J Med* 2005;353(20):2135–47.
24. Chapman PB et al. Improved survival with vemurafenib in melanoma with BRAF V600E mutation. *N Engl J Med* 2011;364(26):2507–16.
25. Hauschild A et al. Dabrafenib in BRAF-mutated metastatic melanoma: A multicentre, open-label, phase 3 randomised controlled trial. *Lancet* 2012;380(9839):358–65.

26. Boussemart L et al. Prospective study of cutaneous side-effects associated with the BRAF inhibitor vemurafenib: A study of 42 patients. *Ann Oncol* 2013;24(6):1691–7.
27. Su F et al. RAS mutations in cutaneous squamous-cell carcinomas in patients treated with BRAF inhibitors. *N Engl J Med* 2012;366(3):207–15.
28. Sinha R, Larkin J, Gore M, Fearfield L. Cutaneous toxicities associated with vemurafenib therapy in 107 patients with BRAF V600E mutation-positive metastatic melanoma, including recognition and management of rare presentations. *Br J Dermatol* 2015;173(4):1024–31.
29. Oberholzer PA et al. RAS mutations are associated with the development of cutaneous squamous cell tumors in patients treated with RAF inhibitors. *J Clin Oncol* 2012;30(3):316–21.
30. Rinderknecht JD et al. RASopathic skin eruptions during vemurafenib therapy. *PLoS One* 2013;8(3):e58721.
31. Holderfield M et al. Vemurafenib cooperates with HPV to promote initiation of cutaneous tumors. *Cancer Res* 2014;74(8):2238–45.
32. Schuurmann M, Ponitzsch I, Simon JC, Ziemer M. Don't miss the base—keratoacanthoma-type squamous cell carcinoma with perineural invasion during BRAF inhibitor therapy for melanoma. *J Dtsch Dermatol Ges* 2015;13(12):1279–81.
33. Braun SA, Gerber PA. Lesion intensified field therapy (LIFT): A new concept in the treatment of actinic field cancerization. *J Eur Acad Dermatol Venereol* 2017;31(5):e232–3.
34. Sachse MM, Wagner G. Clearance of BRAF inhibitor-associated keratoacanthomas by systemic retinoids. *Br J Dermatol* 2014;170(2):475–7.
35. Robert C et al. Improved overall survival in melanoma with combined dabrafenib and trametinib. *N Engl J Med* 2015;372(1):30–39.
36. Sanlorenzo M et al. Comparative profile of cutaneous adverse events: BRAF/MEK inhibitor combination therapy versus BRAF monotherapy in melanoma. *J Am Acad Dermatol* 2014;71(6):1102–1109.e1.
37. Furudate S et al. Keratoacanthoma, palmoplantar keratoderma developing in an advanced melanoma patient treated with vemurafenib regressed by blockade of mitogen-activated protein kinase kinase signaling. *J Dermatol* 2017;44(9):e226–7.
38. Lacouture ME et al. Cutaneous keratoacanthomas/squamous cell carcinomas associated with neutralization of transforming growth factor beta by the monoclonal antibody fresolimumab (GC1008). *Cancer Immunol Immunother* 2015;64(4):437–46.
39. Woodhouse J, Maytin EV. Eruptive nevi of the palms and soles. *J Am Acad Dermatol* 2005;52(5 Suppl 1):S96–S100.
40. Bogenrieder T, Weitzel C, Scholmerich J, Landthaler M, Stolz W. Eruptive multiple lentigo-maligna-like lesions in a patient undergoing chemotherapy with an oral 5-fluorouracil prodrug for metastasizing colorectal carcinoma: A lesson for the pathogenesis of malignant melanoma? *Dermatology* 2002;205(2):174–5.
41. Salopek TG, Mahmood MN. Eruptive melanocytic nevi induced by interferon for nodal metastatic melanoma: Case report and review of the literature. *J Cutan Med Surg* 2013;17(6):410–3.
42. Karrer S, Szeimies RM, Stolz W, Landthaler M. [Eruptive melanocytic nevi after chemotherapy]. *Klin Padiatr* 1998;210(1):43–46.
43. Bovenschen HJ et al. Induction of eruptive benign melanocytic naevi by immune suppressive agents, including biologicals. *Br J Dermatol* 2006;154(5):880–4.
44. Santiago F, Goncalo M, Reis JP, Figueiredo A. Adverse cutaneous reactions to epidermal growth factor receptor inhibitors: A study of 14 patients. *An Bras Dermatol* 2011;86(3):483–90.
45. Chen FW, Tseng D, Reddy S, Daud AI, Swetter SM. Involution of eruptive melanocytic nevi on combination BRAF and MEK inhibitor therapy. *JAMA Dermatol* 2014;150(11):1209–12.
46. Cohen PR, Bedikian AY, Kim KB. Appearance of new vemurafenib-associated melanocytic nevi on normal-appearing skin: Case series and a review of changing or new pigmented lesions in patients with metastatic malignant melanoma after initiating treatment with vemurafenib. *J Clin Aesthet Dermatol* 2013;6(5):27–37.
47. Sibaud V, Munsch C, Lamant L. Eruptive nevi and hair depigmentation related to regorafenib. *Eur J Dermatol* 2015;25(1):85–86.
48. Dalle S, Poulalhon N, Thomas L. Vemurafenib in melanoma with BRAF V600E mutation. *N Engl J Med* 2011;365(15):1448–9; author reply 1450.
49. Curr N, Saunders H, Murugasu A, Cooray P, Schwarz M, Gin D. Multiple periungual pyogenic granulomas following systemic 5-fluorouracil. *Australas J Dermatol* 2006;47(2):130–3.

50. Robert C et al. Nail toxicities induced by systemic anticancer treatments. *Lancet Oncol* 2015;16(4):e181–9.
51. Wollina U. Multiple eruptive periungual pyogenic granulomas during anti-CD20 monoclonal antibody therapy for rheumatoid arthritis. *J Dermatol Case Rep* 2010;4(3):44–46.
52. Sammut SJ, Tomson N, Corrie P. Pyogenic granuloma as a cutaneous adverse effect of vemurafenib. *N Engl J Med* 2014;371(13):1265–7.
53. Groesser L, Peterhof E, Evert M, Landthaler M, Berneburg M, Hafner C. BRAF and RAS mutations in sporadic and secondary pyogenic granuloma. *J Invest Dermatol* 2016;136(2):481–6.
54. Gibney GT, Messina JL, Fedorenko IV, Sondak VK, Smalley KS. Paradoxical oncogenesis—The long-term effects of BRAF inhibition in melanoma. *Nat Rev Clin Oncol* 2013;10(7):390–9.
55. Homey B et al. Escalating therapy of cutaneous side effects of EGFR inhibitors: Experience of German reference centers. *J Dtsch Dermatol Ges* 2012;10(8):559–63.
56. Braam KI et al. Malignant melanoma as second malignant neoplasm in long-term childhood cancer survivors: A systematic review. *Pediatr Blood Cancer* 2012;58(5):665–74.
57. Morton LM et al. Second malignancy risks after non-Hodgkin's lymphoma and chronic lymphocytic leukemia: Differences by lymphoma subtype. *J Clin Oncol* 2010;28(33):4935–44.
58. Hughes BR, Cunliffe WJ, Bailey CC. Excess benign melanocytic naevi after chemotherapy for malignancy in childhood. *BMJ* 1989;299(6691):88–91.
59. Lam CJ et al. Risk factors for melanoma among survivors of non-Hodgkin lymphoma. *J Clin Oncol* 2015;33(28):3096–104.

11

Hypersensitivity and Urticaria

Cataldo Patruno, Maria Ferrillo, and Maria Vastarella

Introduction and Epidemiology

Any administration of an antineoplastic drug can expose a patient to the risk of hypersensitivity reaction (HR); although rarely, severe overreactions can occur. The real frequency of drug hypersensitivity reaction (DHR) is unknown because it is often difficult to prove the relationship between the drug and the reaction; for this reason there is the lack of data on epidemiology of DHR (1). Certain drugs (e.g., taxol) cause reactions with great frequency, while only few antitumor drugs have not had at least one reported instance of causing DHR (2).

Most reactions are immediate (<1 h after the administration), but there are also instances of nonimmediate reactions (>1 h after the administration) caused by many of the antineoplastic agents (3).

The underlying event leading to DHR is a specific sensitization of the immune system to the drug, according to the Gell and Coombs classification of hypersensitivity reactions (Table 11.1).

However, reactions also may arise as a result of nonimmunologic mechanisms and caused by drug intolerance (idiosyncratic or pseudoallergic). Symptoms of a drug-induced pseudoallergic or anaphylactoid reaction resulting from the direct release of histamine and producing flushing, rash, pruritus, urticaria, hypotension, and mucous secretion can sometimes make it difficult to distinguish it from a true DHR. Symptoms are generally more severe in anaphylactic than in anaphylactoid reactions with cardiovascular collapse and bronchospasm occurring more frequently in the former and cutaneous manifestations seen more often in the latter (4).

Among traditional antineoplastic agents, platins and taxanes cause the vast majority of chemotherapy-related HR. In addition during the last decade many new biological immune modulators entered the market as new therapeutic principles for cancer treatment. They comprise proteins such as cytokines, monoclonal antibodies, and fusion proteins (solubilized receptors). HRs are reported also to these drugs, in particular to trastuzumab, panitumumab, rituximab, and cetuximab.

Risk factors for DHR are dependent from patient- and drug-related factors. Patient-related factors are age, gender, (women > men), polymorphisms (HLA, drug-metabolizing enzymes), viral infection (HIV, herpes infections), and cross-reactions (a history of allergic reaction to chemically related drugs or allergic contact dermatitis to chemically related substances). Drug-related factors include molecular size (high-molecular substances or good binding haptens), application, and dosage (Table 11.2).

Diagnosis

The diagnosis of DHR is based on medical history, and *in vivo* and *in vitro* tests (2).

In immediate DHR, the skin prick test is the standard test, followed by intradermal testing if the prick test is negative. Although skin tests are the most accessible means for examining hypersensibility, further study is needed to evaluate their predictive value for HR by chemotherapeutic drugs (5).

Serum IgE measurement is unavailable for most drugs that act as haptens; particularly there are no commercial IgE tests for antineoplastic drugs, but some studies showed their potential use in the diagnosis of HR to platinum-based agents (6). Among *in vitro* tests, the basophil activation test (BAT) is used when skin

TABLE 11.1

Classification of Gell and Coombs

Type	Type of Immune Response	Clinical Features
I	IgE	Urticaria, angioedema, anaphylactic shock, bronchial asthma
II	IgG and FcR	Cytopenia
III	IgG or IgM and complement	Serum sickness, arthus reaction
IVa	Th1	Eczema
IVb	Th2	Maculopapular exanthema, DRESS
IVc	Cytotoxic T cells	Maculopapular exanthema, SJS, TEN
IVd	T cells	Acute generalized exanthematous pustulosis

Abbreviations: DRESS, drug reaction with eosinophilia and systemic symptoms; SJS, Stevens-Johnson syndrome; TEN, toxic epidermal necrolysis.

TABLE 11.2

Risk Factors for DHR

Patient-Related Factors	Drug-Related Factors
Age	Molecular size
Gender	Application
Polymorphisms (HLA, drug-metabolizing enzymes)	Dose
Infections	—
Cross reactions	—

tests and IgE are inconclusive or lacking. BAT evaluates the expression of basophil activation–related proteins (CD63 and CD203c, among others) by flow cytometry after stimulation with the allergen of interest (7).

For nonimmediate DHR, the patch test is the main diagnostic test. There are some risks and contraindications, for example, a history of life-threatening anaphylaxis. On the other hand, the lymphocyte transformation test (LTT), an *in vitro* test measuring memory T-cell response, may be employed, but it is important to perform the test at the right time (8).

In both immediate and nonimmediate reactions, drug provocation test is the gold standard for the identification of DHR, especially when *in vitro* tests are negative, not available, or not validated, taking into account that they have a limited sensitivity (9). It is indicated in a very limited number of cases, particularly when there is clinical evidence of HR against a drug and it is necessary to use that drug in the absence of another drug, not structurally related, equally effective, and when the benefit is most likely above the risk.

Clinical Features

The clinical presentation depends on the drug and mechanism involved. Immediate DHR include urticaria (Figure 11.1), angioedema, bronchospasm, dyspnea, thoracic or abdominal pain, and anaphylaxis, these usually are IgE-mediated reactions and occur during the infusion of the drug (Table 11.3), whereas the clinical picture of nonimmediate reaction is polymorphic and is characterized by, for example, macular and papular eruptions, and vasculitis (Table 11.4) (10).

Immediate reactions can be considered mild, moderate, or severe, and are classified according to Brown's grading system for immediate hypersensitivity reactions. Mild (grade 1) reactions compromise skin and subcutaneous tissues only, whereas moderate (grade 2) and severe (grade 3) reactions may affect cardiovascular, respiratory, and neurological systems (Table 11.5).

Platinum Salts

The platinum salts (oxaliplatin and carboplatin) can cause hypersensitivity reactions with an incidence of over 5%, more often with the immediate type. DHRs usually arise after several infusions, on average

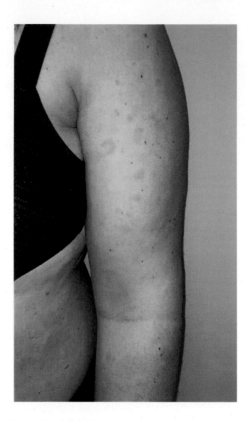

FIGURE 11.1   Acute urticaria during carboplatin therapy.

TABLE 11.3

Clinical Features of Immediate HR to Antineoplastic Drugs

Immediate Reactions	
Anaphylaxis	
Urticarial, angioedema	<1 hour after administration
Exacerbation of asthma	

TABLE 11.4

Clinical Features of Nonimmediate DHR to Antineoplastic Drugs

Nonimmediate Reactions	**Onset**
DRESS, TEN, SJS	>2–6 weeks after administration
AGEP	>3–5 days after administration
Eczema, epatitis, nefritis, photosensitivity	Variable

Abbreviations: AGEP, acute generalized exanthematous pustulosis; DRESS, drug reaction with eosinophilia and systemic symptoms; SJS, Stevens-Johnson syndrome; TEN, toxic epidermal necrolysis.

seven, because there is a need for repeated exposure to the drug to induce an HR. There are conflicting data in the literature on estimated prevalence of adverse reactions (5).

Oxaliplatin is associated with 0.5–25% of mild to moderate HR, but also with 1% of life-threatening adverse events. In the most of cases, HRs occur at the end or shortly after the end of infusion and improved with intravenous antihistamines and steroids treatment. Premedication schedules have not been completely reliable in preventing oxaliplatin reactions, and desensitization protocols should be considered (6).

TABLE 11.5

Brown's Grading System for Immediate Hypersensitivity Reactions

Grade	Severity	Description
1	Mild	Symptoms limited to the skin (e.g., flushing) or involve a single organ/system and are mild
2	Moderate	Symptoms involve at least two organs/systems (e.g., flushing and dyspnea) and are mild, but there is no significant drop in blood pressure or in oxygen saturation
3	Severe	Symptoms involve at least two organs/systems (e.g., flushing and dyspnea) and there is a significant drop in blood pressure and/or in oxygen saturation

For carboplatin, about 50% of the reactions occur near to the end of administration, showing a long time to resolution and arising after a median of five cycles and poorly responding to antihistamines or steroids (4). An HR is a potentially lethal adverse event that frequently requires discontinuation of the drug. The risk of reaction is supposed to be associated with a previous history of drug allergy, a prolonged platinum-free interval, or high dosages of carboplatin. Intradermal injections of carboplatin can be used to predict carboplatin-induced severe DHRs (7).

For diagnosis of reactions induced by platinum salts, IgE tests present sensitivity less than that of skin testing but high specificity. A major advantage of this test is the ability to detect IgE shortly after the reactions than without the need to wait several weeks to determine skin test reactivity, which can damage the cancer response to chemotherapy. Another advantage is the finding of cross-reactivity, which is seen in patients reactive to oxaliplatin with specific IgE for oxaliplatin, carboplatin, and cisplatin (11).

Taxanes

Taxanes (paclitaxel and docetaxel) are an important cause of hypersensitivity reactions in cancer patients. Three factors were identified as predictive factors: younger age, a history of allergy, and short-course premedication (12). As already reported in the literature, taxane-associated DHRs are dose and rate dependent. Previous studies suggested that HR to paclitaxel and docetaxel are primarily due to a type I reaction to the pharmaceutical vehicle, called cremophor, used to solubilize paclitaxel. However recent findings have raised the possibility that some of these DHR are IgE-mediated.

Literature data reports a higher incidence of adverse reactions with paclitaxel compared with docetaxel. In an Italian case series (11), 98 HRs occurred with taxanes (87/240 paclitaxel; 11/240 docetaxel). Paclitaxel had an incidence of 1.2% (87 of 7360 paclitaxel administrations) as did docetaxel (11 of 912 docetaxel infusions).

Most of HRs caused by taxanes occur at infusion beginning (Figure 11.2), generally after the first or second drug exposure (13). Reactions were seen at the beginning of treatment both with paclitaxel (87%) and with docetaxel (100%) (11). These reactions usually occur quite rapidly, which were similar to DHRs caused by contrast media. It seems difficult to reconcile the fact that most patients react upon the first or second exposure (leaving a little opportunity for sensitization) with an IgE-mediated mechanism. This mystery could potentially be explained by the fact that sensitivity to taxanes can develop without exposure to the drug, possibly via airbone exposure. Indeed paclitaxel and the precursors for docetaxel (baccatin III and 3-deacetylbaccatin III) have been isolated from different species of yew trees and from different parts of the plant including its pollen, and these could explain why DHRs are more common in atopic subjects (14).

Appropriate premedication management is extremely important to prevent reactions. Without premedication, DHRs are reported in 30% of patients, whereas with standard medications the incidence falls to <4%. Paclitaxel premedication consisted of oral administration of prednisone, 25 mg 12 h before, and of hydrocortisone (250 mg) + chlorphenamine (10 mg) + ranitidine (50 mg) iv, given 30 min before drug infusion. In regard to docetaxel premedication, it consisted of oral administration of dexamethasone at the dosage of 4 mg for 3 days, starting 1 day before chemotherapy, and of dexamethasone, 8 mg intravenously on the day of therapy.

Recently, a novel paclitaxel formulation, nab-paclitaxel, was formed. Nanoparticle albumin-bound paclitaxel (nab-paclitaxel) does not contain Cremophor EL. It uses human serum albumin to encapsulate

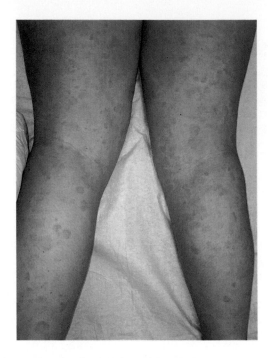

FIGURE 11.2   Hypersensitivity reaction after first infusions of docetaxel.

hydrophobic paclitaxel molecules in particles of around 130 nm. Nab-paclitaxel in contrast to the other taxanes does not require the use of premedication to prevent DHR (15). Most taxane-induced reactions are immediate, and the signs and symptoms are thought to be the result of basophil/mast cell degranulation. Although less common than immediate DHRs, a range of delayed, possibly immune-mediated, reactions have been described with taxanes. Importantly, delayed onset skin eruptions (most commonly a benign maculopapular rash) can be the prelude to an immediate DHR during the next infusion. Stevens-Johnson syndrome (SJS) and toxic epidermal necrolysis (TEN) have also been described (17).

Taxane skin testing, which identifies patients with an IgE-mediated sensitivity, appears as a promising diagnostic and risk stratification tool in the management of patients with DHR to taxanes. Skin testing should be performed at least 2 weeks after the event to minimize the possibility of a false-negative result due to the refractory period following a DHR (17).

Targeted Therapies

Monoclonal antibodies are innovative drugs used to treat different human diseases. Although designed to be significantly more "precise" than traditional chemotherapies, targeted therapies frequently induce DHRs. Hypersensitivity reactions have been reported for all monoclonal antibodies, especially with trastuzumab, panitumumab, rituximab, and cetuximab.

In general, the incidence of DHR varies from 15 to 20% for cetuximab (3% grade 3–4) and 40% for trastuzumab (<1% grade 3–4) to 77% for rituximab (10% grade 3–4) (16). Even after the fourth infusion, 30% of cancer patients react to rituximab, and the incidence of DHR remains 14% after the eighth infusion. Approximately 80% of fatal reactions occurred after the first rituximab infusion.

Furthermore most HRs to cetuximab occur within minutes after the first exposure to the drug and are associated with IgE antibodies against GA lactose-α-1,3-galactose (17). Galactose-a-1,3-galactose is in the Fab portion of the cetuximab heavy chain (18). Reactions to cetuximab seem to be mediated by an identical mechanism of red meat allergy, related to oligosaccharides in the meat (19). Premedication with a minimum dose of betamethasone might prevent most hypersensitivity reactions to cetuximab (20).

Delayed hypersensitivity reactions to biologicals have been reported, with reports of rash, serum sickness–like symptoms, vasculitis, erythema multiforme, Stevens-Johnson syndrome, and toxic epidermal necrolysis. When a patient presents a hypersensitivity reaction to a biological, rapid desensitization is a groundbreaking procedure that will enable the patient to receive the full treatment dose while protecting him from anaphylaxis (17).

Immunotherapy

Antibodies that target key immune checkpoints, such as cytotoxic T-lymphocyte antigen-4 (ipilimumab) and programmed death-1 (pembrolizumab and nivolumab), have emerged as clinically effective treatment options for melanoma and other tumor types, including non-small cell lung cancer and renal cell carcinoma. Rash, pruritus, and vitiligo were the most frequently reported skin adverse events. The calculated incidence of all-grade rash with pembrolizumab and nivolumab was 16.7% and 14.3%, respectively. The onset, ranged widely (3 weeks to 2 years), which may be indicative of both an acute and delayed immunological reaction to these drugs, as seen with many other drug-induced skin eruptions.

The rashes generally manifest with erythematous macules, papules, and plaques, predominantly localized to the trunk and extremities, and may be associated with pruritus. Maculopapular eruptions are responsive to low-potency topical corticosteroids (21).

Management and Conclusions

Numerous therapeutic agents are available for the treatment of oncologic diseases. These drugs have achieved great improvements in clinical outcomes. On the other hand, many kinds of adverse reactions are observed in patients undergoing both traditional and targeted treatments. These reactions might greatly influence the therapeutic strategy. Among adverse drug reactions, allergic reactions remain common and are often underdiagnosed. Moderate to severe hypersensitivity reactions usually require cessation of therapy or the replacement of the drug, which largely interferes with improved patient management. Several options are available based on the severity of the DHR and the therapeutic alternatives such as definitive discontinuation, premedication measures, or desensitization protocols. In particular, drug desensitization should be considered standard of care when patients need first-line therapy (11). The management of patients following a DHR involves risk stratification, and reexposure could be performed either through rapid drug desensitization or graded challenge based on the severity of the initial DHR and the skin test result.

In literature there are several desensitization protocols, but the diversity and sometimes-conflicting nature of the data show the need to validate desensitization protocols in a large number of patients, which includes patients with severe DHRs and ideally in different populations to reliably establish their safety and efficacy.

Rapid drug desensitization has been shown to be an effective and safe method to reintroduce taxanes in hundreds of patients, including those with life-threatening DHRs. Patients with nonsevere delayed skin DHRs may benefit from rapid drug desensitization since they may be at increased risk for an immediate DHR upon reexposure.

Usually short lasting, this kind of reaction does not require any specific treatment in most cases or, if not successful, prompt administration of steroids is enough to control the symptoms. Intensive care unit intervention is rarely required (11).

REFERENCES

1. Demoly P et al. International Consensus on drug allergy. *Allergy* 2014;69:420–37.
2. Raymond B et al. Hypersensitivity reactions from antineoplastic agents. *Cancer Metastasis Rev* 1987;6:413–32.
3. Giavina-Bianchi P et al. Immediate hypersensitivity reaction to chemotherapeutic agents. *J Allergy Clin Immunol* 2017;5:593–9.
4. Brian A et al. Adverse reactions to targeted and non-targeted chemotherapeutic drugs with emphasis on hypersensitivity responses and the invasive metastatic switch. *Cancer Metastasis Rev* 2013;32:723–61.

5. Patil SU et al. A protocol for risk stratification of patients with carboplatin-induced hypersensitivity reactions. *J Allergy Clin Immunol* 2012;129:443–7.

6. Madrigal-Burgaleta R et al. Hypersensitivity and desensitization to antineoplastic agents: Outcomes of 189 procedures with a new short protocol and novel diagnostic tools assessment. *Allergy* 2013;68:853–61.

7. Song WJ et al. Recent applications of basophil activation tests in the diagnosis of drug hypersensitivity. *Asia Pacific Allergy* 2013;3:266–80.

8. Baldo B et al. Adverse reactions to targeted and non-targeted chemotherapeutic drugs with emphasis on hypersensitivity responses and the invasive metastatic switch. *Cancer Metastasis Rev* 2013;32:723–61.

9. Demoly P et al. Determining the negative predictive value of provocation tests with beta-lactams. *Allergy* 2010;65:327–32.

10. Ferrari L et al. Are antineoplastic drug acute hypersensitive reactions a submerged or an emergent problem? Experience of the Medical Day Hospital of the Fondazione IRCCS IstitutoNazionaleTumori. *Tumori* 2014;100:9–14.

11. Castells M et al. Diagnosis and management of anaphylaxis in precision medicine. *J Allergy Clin Immunol* 2017;140:321–33.

12. Aoyama T et al. Is there any predictor for hypersensitivity reactions in gynecologic cancer patients treated with paclitaxel-based therapy? *Cancer Chemother Pharmacol* 2017;80:65–9. Epub 2017 May 10.

13. Markman M et al. Paclitaxel-associated hypersensitivity reactions: Experience of the gynecologic oncology program of the Cleveland Clinic Cancer Center. *J Clin Oncol* 2000;18:102–5.

14. Vanhaelen M et al. Taxanes in *Taxus baccata* pollen: Cardiotoxicity and/or allergenicity? *Planta Med* 2002;68:36–40.

15. Picard M et al. Re-visiting hypersensitivity reactions to Taxanes: A comprehensive review. *Clin Rev Allergy Immunol* 2015;49:177–91.

16. Galvão et al. Hypersensitivity to biological agents-updated diagnosis, management, and treatment. *J Allergy Clin Immunol Pract* 2015;3:175–85; quiz 186.

17. Chung CH et al. Cetuximab-induced anaphylaxis and IgE specific for galactose-alpha-1,3-galactose. *N Engl J Med* 2008;358:1109–17.

18. Munoz-Cano et al. Biological agents: New drugs, old problems. *J Allergy Clin Immunol* 2010;126:394–95.

19. Saleh H et al. Anaphylactic reactions to oligosaccharides in red meat: A syndrome in evolution. *Clin Mol Allergy* 2012;10:5.

20. Ikegawa K et al. Retrospective analysis of premedication, glucocorticosteroids, and H1-antihistamines for preventing infusion reactions associated with cetuximab treatment of patients with head and neck cancer. *J Int Med Res* 2017;45:1378–85.

21. Belum VR et al. Characterization and management of dermatologic adverse events to agents targeting the PD-1 receptor. *Eur J Cancer* 2016;60:12–25.

12

Xerosis, Itching, and Fissures

Gabriella Fabbrocini, Tiziana Peduto, and Mariateresa Cantelli

EGFR/Ligand System and Maintenance of the Epidermal Barrier

Normal skin architecture is dramatically perturbed by epidermal growth factor receptor (EGFR) inhibition, with loss of basal cell proliferative potential and perturbed keratinocyte differentiation. Epidermal upper layers are compromised too, due to reduced tight junction proteins. The formation and function of the stratum corneum is eventually lost, with increased desquamation; loss of body fluid; and facilitated access of environmental microbes, particles, and chemicals. Such defects in host defense mechanisms may lead to microbial invasion and frequent skin infections. We repeatedly noticed that epidermis deprived of EGFR signaling may lead to deranged expression and release of crucial chemokines and cytokines with consequent massive recruitment and activation of immune cell populations, and eventual manifestation of skin damage (1).

As it has been amply illustrated, a synergistic interplay exists between EGFR activation and the mechanism of innate immunity in the human skin in order to maximally enhance AMP expression: Inhibition of the EGFR blocks both the neutrophilic chemotactic activity and the expression of the majority of the AMPs. This defect leads to dry, scaly, and strongly itchy skin, with subsequent dehydration (2).

EGFR Inhibitor Agents: Skin–Mucous Toxicity

EGFR inhibitor (EGFRi) use involves the onset of toxicity at the level of tissue regions, whose function is strictly dependent on EGFR and EGFR-mediated signaling (3).

The major secondary side effect of using EGFRis is strongly felt in the skin–mucous region, where EGFR is constitutively expressed in the keratinocytes of the basal epidermis layer, the outer sheath of the hair follicle, the sebaceous glands, and the sweat glands eccrine, which on the clinical plane is extrinsic with rash, papulo-pustulosis, skin xerosis, alteration of hair growth, itching, nausea, and, less frequently, hyperpigmentation, trichomegaly, telangiectasia, and mucositis.

Skin toxicity plays a key role in the patient's quality of life, affecting the physical, psychological, and social well-being of the individual, and may be so impactful as to lead to discontinuation or dose reduction of the drug. Therefore, an appropriate therapeutic approach to this toxicity appears to be absolutely necessary in order to achieve a balance between administering the drug, improving the patient's quality of life, and patient outcomes (3). In particular, skin xerosis affects more than 80% of patients who are using EGFR inhibitors (4). Advanced age, atopy, and previous cytotoxic agents are the most commonly promoted factors. Dry skin, or xerosis, usually begins between the first and second months of therapy. By 3 months, 50% of patients are affected, and by 6 months 100% of those who receive EGFR-targeted therapy will experience a degree of xerosis (5). This may manifest as dry skin, asteatotic dermatitis, or, in severe cases, skin splitting or fissuring (5). It is typically presented with dry, desquamated, pruriginous skin, and generally involves the same areas previously affected by acneiform eruption (face, trunk, ends) (Figure 12.1).

Dryness can progressively evolve into a real eczema and worsen in secondary infections by *Staphylococcus aureus*, or more rarely by herpesvirus. Sometimes it may also appear in the form of a

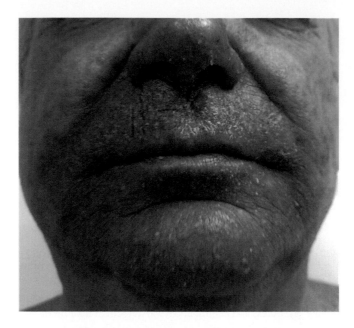

FIGURE 12.1 Desquamated and dry skin involving the face in a patient treated with anti-EGFR.

dry, painful pulp to the fingertips of the fingers and toes, often associated with painful fissures at the fingertips, nail folds, and interphalangeal joints (Figure 12.2) (6).

The skin tends to thinner, resulting in increased skin fragility and the chance to detect, in such patients, bruising in the most affected areas (4). Reguiai et al. divided xerosis in three different degrees of severity as follows: grade 1, slight, <10% of the body surface area without related erythema or pruritus; grade 2, moderate, >10% and <30% of the body surface area with related erythema or pruritus, and limiting key

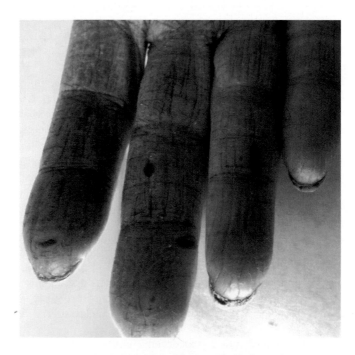

FIGURE 12.2 Dry skin and fissures at the fingertips in patient treated with anti-EGFR.

daily routine activities (food preparation, using the telephone, etc.); grade 3, severe, affecting over 30% of the body surface area with related erythema or pruritus, and limiting key daily routine activities in the specific management of the patient (washing oneself, taking medication, etc.) (7).

It should also be taken into consideration that dryness can also occur in the mucous membranes, especially the vaginal, and the perineum, with discomfort during urination. Skin xerosis predisposes to the onset of itching, a symptom almost entirely reported by patients. It is usually generalized and exacerbated by heat, and presents at day and at night causing an interrupted sleep. There is often no primary rash; however, there may be numerous linear excoriations on the skin secondary to scratching (5). It tends to persist even after the suspension of the therapy (8). The pathogenesis of xerosis is linked to the alteration of skin barrier integrity highlighted during therapy with EGFRis. Indeed, numerous studies have shown that knock-out mice for EGFR tend to develop drier skin, with decreasing production of loricrin in the granular epidermis layer. This molecule plays a key role in maintaining the epidermis barrier function, as it represents the most abundant protein of the stratum corneum, which, in addition to serving as an important barrier protein, also contributes to counteract transepidermal water loss and electrolysis (4).

Therapeutic Management of Cutaneous Toxicity

General Prophylactic Measures

Prior to initiating EGFRi therapy, each candidate patient should undergo a careful medical history, assisted by objective examination, with the aim of highlighting recent or current xerosis, acne vulgaris, or atopic dermatitis. In addition, in order to reduce the risk of skin toxicity, it is necessary for patients with anti-EGFR therapy to

1. Use, for personal care, nonaggressive detergents and avoid the use of alcohol-containing products such as lotions or perfumes that can cause irritation and exacerbate xerosis.
2. Avoid the use of synthetic garments, before resorting to natural fibers, and avoid wearing too-tight shoes.
3. Use moisturizing baths and creams to keep skin hydrated and keep bathing time short.
4. Limit sun exposure and use highly protective sunscreens year-round (sun protection factor [SPF] greater than 30), preferring the physical filters containing zinc oxide or titanium dioxide.

Therapeutic Strategies Specific to Any Type of Skin Toxicity

The side effects found during therapy with EGFRis can be approached through topical or systemic treatments; the choice of one or other therapy is dictated by the type and severity of the clinic. It is essential to educate and instruct the patient to recognize and report in a timely manner any possible signs of toxicity in order to be able to intervene early and to ensure a better outcome.

To reduce skin dryness, it is important to follow general prophylactic measures and the daily use of emollient creams/balms even in occlusion, and avoid too frequent and aggressive detergents. A widespread erythema associated with an important pruritus may be significant therefore, requiring the use of medium-dose topical corticosteroids for 1–2 weeks (betamethasone-propionate 0.05% cream, flucinolone acetonide ointment or hydrocortisone butyrate 0.1% cream).

In case of secondary overcapacity for scratching, it is recommended to use topical antibiotics such as 2% fusidic acid, bacitracin cream, or 2% mupirocin cream. If eczema and desquamation exhibit grade 3 severity, the use of systemic steroids is preferred in order to avoid the evolution into a severe form of exfoliative dermatitis (grade 4 toxicity).

Xerosis is generally associated with itchiness, which must be treated with either urea- or polidocanol-based emollients, as well as with first-generation H1 antihistamines, such as cetirizine, loratadine, fexofenadine, and ebastine.

Fractures can be treated with occlusive and hydrocolloid dressings, pedicures/manicures with antiseptic solutions (0.025% potassium permanganate), and topical applications of silver nitrate solutions to accelerate healing. The use of base creams of urea applied on the peripheral skin tends both to favor cicatrization and to prevent the onset.

REFERENCES

1. Pastore S, Lulli D, Girolomoni G. Epidermal growth factor receptor signalling in keratinocyte biology: Implications for skin toxicity of tyrosine kinase inhibitors. *Arch Toxicol* 2014;88(6):1189–203.
2. Pastore S, Mascia F, Mariani V, Girolomoni G. The epidermal growth factor receptor system in skin repair and inflammation. *J Invest Dermatol* 2008;128:1365–74.
3. Hu JC et al. Cutaneous side effects of epidermal growth factor receptor inhibitors: Clinical presentation, pathogenesis and management. *J Am Acad Dermatol* 2007;56:317–26.
4. Segaert S, van Cutsem E. Clinical signs, pathophysiology and management of skin toxicity during therapy with epidermal growth factor receptor inhibitors. *Ann Oncol* 2005;16:1425–33.
5. Sinclair R. Anticipating and managing the cutaneous side effects of epidermal growth factor receptor inhibitors. *Asia Pac J Clin Oncol* Mar 2014;10 Suppl 1:11–7.
6. Busam KJ et al. Cutaneous side-effects in patients treated with the antiepidermal growth factor receptor antibody C225. *Br J Dermatol* 2001;144:1169–76.
7. Reguiai Z et al. Management of cutaneous adverse events induced by anti-EGFR (epidermal growth factor receptor): A French interdisciplinary therapeutic algorithm. *Support Care Cancer* 2012;20(7):1395–404.
8. Threadgill DW et al. Targeted disruption of mouse EGF receptor: Effect of genetic background on mutant phenotype. *Science* 1995;269:230–4.

13

Radiation Dermatitis

John David Strickley and Jae Yeon Jung

Terminology

The *gray* (Gy) is the absorption of one joule of ionizing radiation per kilogram of mass. It is the standard unit of measure of radiation dose. 1 Gy $= 1$ J/kg $= 100$ rad $= 100$ cGy

Dose fractionation divides the total dose into smaller doses that are separated by time. This strategy allows for a higher total dose of radiation while minimizing toxicity to normal tissues.

Boost is the use of additional radiation on top of a normal dosing schedule for enhanced tumor control.

Introduction

Because radiotherapy has only modest specificity for malignant cells, normal cells along its path will always be damaged. The skin is the most common unwanted victim to radiotherapy's powerful cellular toxicity. Up to 95% of patients will develop erythema, a type of acute radiation dermatitis, following a one-time exposure to 8 grays (Gy) of radiation (1). Exposures of 70 Gy can lead to skin necrosis in 50% of patients (2).

Although the skin is often a bystander to the toxic effects of radiation therapy, in some diseases the skin is the target. Radiotherapy in cutaneous disease is commonly indicated in the treatment of nonmelanoma skin cancer (Figure 13.1), but also in cutaneous T-cell lymphoma, angiosarcoma, Merkel cell carcinoma, and others. One of the most critical elements of an effective treatment strategy is the choice of modality. The most commonly used modality in dermatology is external beam radiation. Others include brachytherapy, total skin electron beam (TSEB), intensity modulated radiotherapy (IMRT), and stereotactic body radiation therapy (SBRT), and each of these has different roles depending on the disease process and patient characteristics.

External beam radiation therapy uses ionizing radiation in the form of photons (X-rays or gamma rays) or charged particles (electrons or protons). Contemporary external beam radiation employs a linear accelerator to electrically generate X-rays (more simply referred to as photons) or electrons, with the former being the most preferred modality in skin cancer treatment (3). Traditional brachytherapy is the direct application of a radioactive source, rather than electronic, via a surface applicator or catheters. Newer developments include the use of electronic, isotope-free brachytherapy (Xoft®). TSEB exposes the entire skin surface to ionizing electrons and is used in cutaneous T-cell lymphoma. The introduction of IMRT was an extremely important step toward reducing damage to normal tissue. This image-guided modality uses a collimator to contour the radiation beam to the shape of the malignancy, and then radiates from multiple angles in order to disperse the dose delivered to normal tissue. Another major advancement was SBRT, which was a form of extracranial stereotactic radiosurgery that compensates for movement of target tissue during beam delivery. To do so, SBRT utilizes in-room imaging to adjust for patient breathing and other movements, again, with the goal of minimizing dose to normal tissues (4).

Dose fractionation is among the most important strategies of increasing the radiosensitivity of malignant cells relative to normal tissue. This strategy takes advantage of certain biologic qualities of tumor cells (proliferation, cell cycle phase, repair capacity, and oxygenation) in order to increase malignant cell kill and decrease detriment to normal tissues (4). Determination of fractionation schedules is in part guided

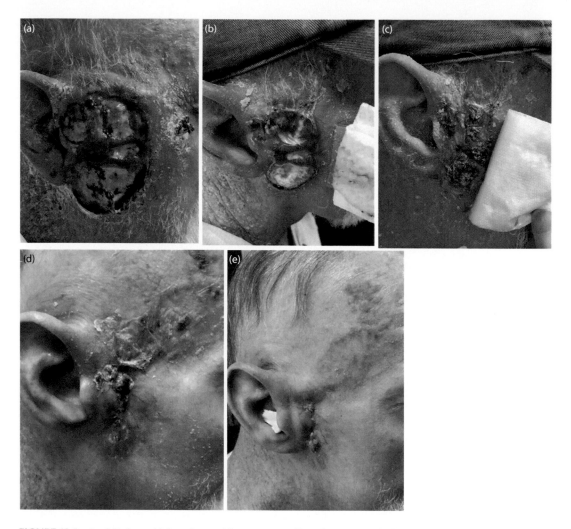

FIGURE 13.1 (a–e) Patient with large inoperable squamous cell carcinoma treated primarily with radiation. He developed multiple complications including acute radiation dermatitis with both dry and wet desquamation. He also developed features of chronic radiation dermatitis with alopecia, fibrosis, and telangiectasia.

by the α/β ratio of a given tumor; most tumors have high α/β ratios, and thus respond to more fractions with lower dosages. As discussed later, this fractionation schedule is ideal because it decreases the risk of acute and chronic skin toxicities.

Mechanism of Action

Ionizing radiation causes molecules to eject an electron, which leads to the production of highly reactive free radicals. The most important cellular target of radiation is DNA (4). Direct interaction of radiation with cellular DNA can result in loss of an electron, thus ionization. This direct interaction between DNA and radiation is termed "direct radiation action." Indirect radiation action occurs when free radicals (e.g., the hydroxyl radical) are formed following radiolysis of water, which then go on to ionize DNA (5). Water is the most abundant molecule in the cell, and, correspondingly, indirect radiation action is an essential contributor to DNA damage.

Possession of an unpaired electron causes molecules to undergo deleterious transmutations in an effort to establish stability. In the case of DNA, these transmutations can lead to strand breakage, nucleotide loss, nucleotide dimerization, and more (3). Mitotic catastrophe, apoptosis, necrosis, and senescence are all common modes of cell death following radiation (6). In some cases, radiation-induced cell death leads to an antitumor immune response. This phenomenon, called the abscopal effect, results in regression of untreated metastases and may be enhanced by immunomodulating cancer therapies (e.g., ipilimumab) (7).

Radiation Dermatitis

Acute Radiation Dermatitis

Acute radiation dermatitis (Figures 13.2 through 13.5) is the most common manifestation of radiation toxicity of the skin and occurs in well over 70% of patients undergoing radiotherapy for cancer (8). The skin's response to radiation varies depending on patient factors (e.g., preexisting conditions) and treatment factors (e.g., dose, site, and fractionation). The pathophysiology is multifactorial, with major contributions from radiation-induced inflammation, direct damage of radiosensitive skin cells, and disrupted wound healing (9,10).

Acute radiation dermatitis is graded based on clinical evaluation of severity (grades 1–5); a commonly used grading system is the Common Terminology Criteria for Adverse Events (CTCAE) (11) (https://evs.nci.nih.gov/ftp1/CTCAE/CTCAE_4.03_2010-06-14). Grade 1 changes include faint erythema or dry desquamation. A patient with grade 2 radiation dermatitis has moderate to brisk erythema, patchy moist desquamation mostly confined to skin folds or creases, and moderate edema. Grade 3 is heralded by moist desquamation in areas other than skin folds or creases and bleeding with minor abrasions. A skin graft is indicated in grade 4, which denotes the presence of necrosis or full-thickness ulceration (Figure 13.5) and spontaneous bleeding. Last, grade 5 is death.

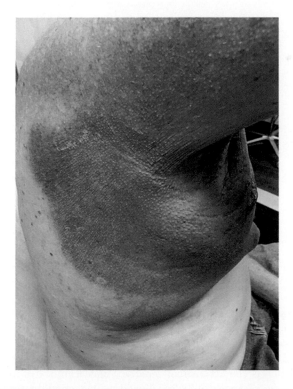

FIGURE 13.2 Acute radiation dermatitis. Patient with metastatic melanoma undergoing radiation treatment for large axillary tumor. Note well-demarcated erythema and areas of dry desquamation. He complained of slight pruritus without tenderness.

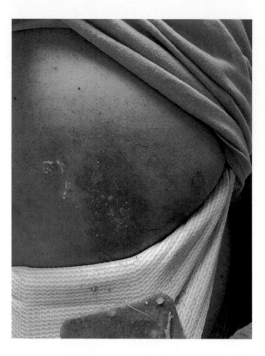

FIGURE 13.3 Acute radiation dermatitis. Patient with metastatic lung cancer with acute radiation dermatitis. Note superficial erosions (wet desquamation). She was complaining of pain and pruritus.

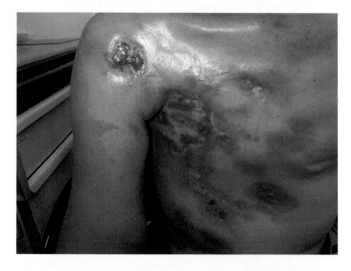

FIGURE 13.4 Acute radiation dermatitis. Patient with breast cancer treated with mastectomy and a prolonged course of radiation. She developed erosions and underlying fibrosis.

Preventive measures include skin care practices such as gentle washing with mild soap and emollient moisturizer. There is evidence supporting the use of preventive topical corticosteroids (12). Treatment of grade 1 reactions includes emollient moisturizers, as sebaceous and eccrine glands lose functionality; patients should clean the irradiated area between radiation treatments, as it can reduce bacterial load. Moist desquamation, which is characteristic of grades 2 and 3, indicates increased susceptibility to infection, thus therapy includes the use of hydrocolloid dressings or antibacterial silver-based dressings (13,14); if a secondary infection is suspected, a skin swab from the affected area should be performed. Grade 4 reactions may require debridement, skin grafting, and discontinuation of radiotherapy.

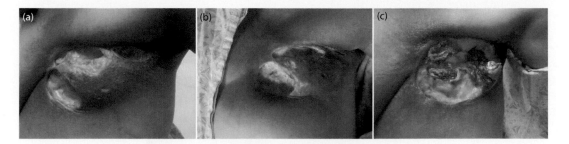

FIGURE 13.5 Patient with breast cancer treated primarily with low-dose radiation for 7 months: (a,b) July; (c) October of the same year. She developed progressive necrosis and ultimately presented with desiccated exposed ribs.

Secondary Infection

Acute radiation dermatitis can lead to persistent nonhealing ulcerations, desquamation, bullae, hemorrhage, and necrosis. Chronic radiation dermatitis can also cause open wounds, all of which pose an increased risk of infection. Secondary infection, namely, with *Staphylococcus aureus* (Figure 13.6) due to its capacity to produce superantigens, has been suggested to intensify the inflammatory processes of radiation toxicity (15). It can be managed like other skin and soft tissue infections with systemic and/ or topical antibiotics.

Chronic Radiation Dermatitis

The manifestations of chronic radiation dermatitis occur months to years following completion of radiotherapy. These changes are also referred to as "late-stage" reactions and may occur in skin that appears otherwise normal following therapy. The incidence of chronic radiation dermatitis is related to total dose and is even more severe if given in high-dose fractions (e.g., 2.5 Gy or higher) (16–18).

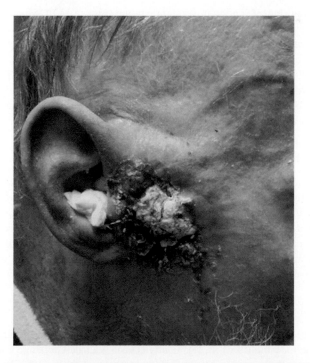

FIGURE 13.6 Patient with large, neglected cutaneous SCC presenting with secondary staphylococcus infection. He presented with pain, tenderness, and malodorous drainage. Surrounding areas show erythema and dry desquamation.

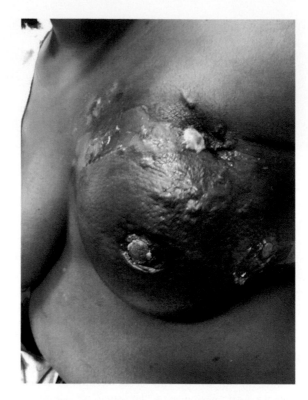

FIGURE 13.7   Chronic radiation dermatitis. Postinflammatory hyperpigmentation following radiation therapy for breast cancer. She also developed dermal edema (peau d'orange) with breast heaviness and pain.

One common late-stage manifestation is dyspigmentation (Figure 13.7), which is commonly a result of postinflammatory changes in epithelial regeneration. Dyspigmentation may also occur as an early-stage reaction. Similarly, necrosis is a feature of both acute (Figure 13.5) and chronic reactions (see Figure 13.10). Alopecia (Figures 13.1e and 13.8) and anhidrosis occur secondary to the exquisite radiosensitivity of the hair follicle and eccrine sweat glands (Figure 13.9), respectively (19). These changes can also occur acutely. Skin atrophy is a late-stage change that occurs secondary to radiation-induced vascular damage and alterations in fibroblasts (14). Other possible chronic, or late-stage, changes will be presented individually. These features are often overlapping.

Radiation-Induced Fibrosis

Fibrosis of irradiated normal tissues (e.g., skin, lungs, and gut) is a late-stage reaction with significant functional and cosmetic sequelae (Figures 13.10 through 13.12). Radiation-induced fibrosis (RIF) is largely cytokine-mediated, with major contributions from TGF-β (20). Radiation also induces terminal differentiation of fibroblast progenitor cells leading to a population of profibrotic atypical fibrocytes (21). Pharmacologic treatment of RIF aims to block inflammatory pathways and free radical damage. Regimens include intramuscular superoxide dismutase or pentoxifylline alone or in combination with vitamin E (22,23). Physical therapy and massage may also be considered (24).

Telangiectasia

The presence of telangiectasia in irradiated skin has historically been used as an endpoint to study the incidence of chronic radiodermatitis (2,18,25). Telangiectasia is a true late-stage finding (Figure 13.13); its appearance occurs in months to years with continuous progression thereafter (17). Both its incidence and latency are dose-dependent, with larger doses and fractions leading to increased incidence and decreased

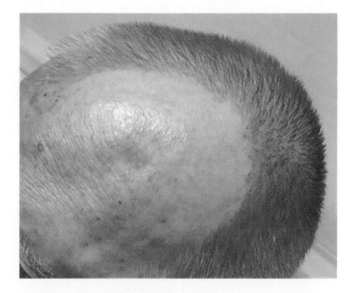

FIGURE 13.8 Chronic radiation dermatitis. Patient with atypical fibroxanthoma of the scalp treated with radiation. The treatment area is apparent with the well-demarcated patch of alopecia.

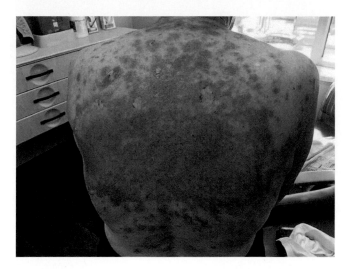

FIGURE 13.9 Chronic radiation dermatitis. Patient with non-small cell lung cancer treated with concurrent radiation and chemotherapy (cisplatin and pemetrexed). She developed lupus-like drug reaction sparing the radiated site, presumably due to loss of adnexal structures.

latency (17). Fifty percent of patients will develop telangiectasia within 5 years following exposure to 65 Gy (2). Although the true pathogenesis is unknown, it is assumed to be related to ionizing radiation's propensity to damage endothelium as well as generate microthrombi. Conflicting data have shown a correlation with the early-stage finding of moist desquamation, which suggests damage to the superficial capillary plexus as a possible mechanism for this late-stage finding (25). Pulsed dye laser treatment has been shown to be an effective therapy (26).

Radiation Recall

Radiation recall dermatitis is an adverse drug reaction that is always confined within the borders of formerly irradiated skin (Figure 13.14). The typical reaction is in response to a chemotherapeutic, occurs within days of introduction of the drug, and within months following cessation of radiotherapy (27).

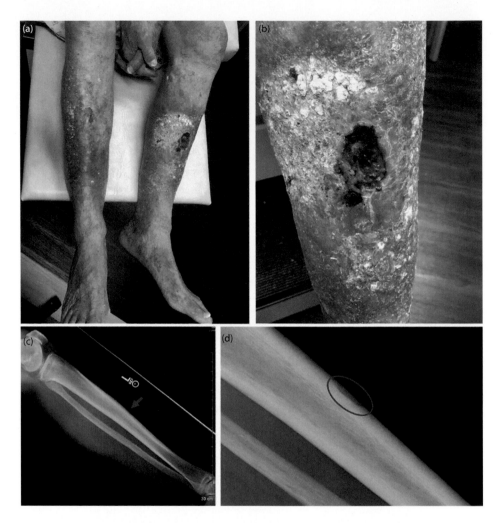

FIGURE 13.10 Chronic radiation dermatitis. Patient with recurrent squamous cell carcinoma of the lower leg treated with radiation. He had numerous varicosities and poor healing (a). The treatments were completed 2 years prior to presentation. He developed progressive fibrosis of the left leg with woody induration and persistent scaling (b). The ulceration resulted in underlying bone erosion (c,d) consistent with radiation necrosis.

Radiation recall dermatitis shares many characteristics of acute radiation dermatitis in that its severity is variable and it may present with erythema, edema, vesiculation, necrosis, and ulceration (14). Urticarial-like lesions may also be seen. The etiology of radiation recall is unknown and the role of treatment, such as topical corticosteroids, is unclear (27). The reaction is managed by dose reduction or cessation of the offending agent.

Edema/Mastitis

Edema is a major acute and chronic manifestation of radiation. Edema in the acute setting is likely secondary to radiation-induced inflammation, microthrombi, and endothelial damage. In the breast, the risk of chronic edema may be increased by factors such as irradiated breast volume and the dose of a photon boost (28). Common clinical findings include peau d'orange, breast heaviness, erythema, pain, skin thickening, hyperpigmentation, and pitting (Figures 13.7 and 13.15) (29). Of particular interest, the clinical finding peau d'orange may arouse suspicion of a secondary malignancy (e.g., inflammatory carcinoma) leading to unnecessary testing.

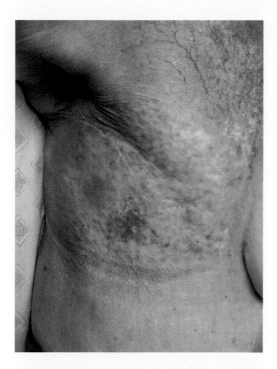

FIGURE 13.11 Chronic radiation dermatitis. Patient with breast cancer treated with mastectomy and radiation. Skin developed fibrosis that was bound down and restricted her range of motion. She developed extensive telangiectatic vessels.

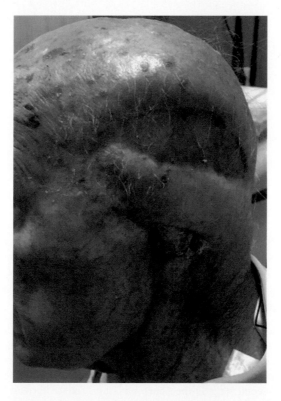

FIGURE 13.12 Patient with multiple recurrent cutaneous squamous cell carcinoma. He was treated with wide local excision, neck dissection, skin graft, and radiation. Chronic fibrotic changes with exposed temporal bone.

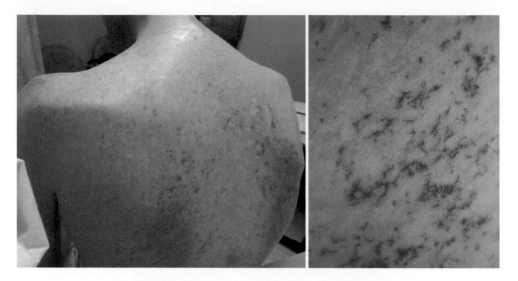

FIGURE 13.13   Patient with non-Hodgkin's lymphoma treated with hematopoietic cell transplant. He received total body irradiation and developed extensive telangiectasias.

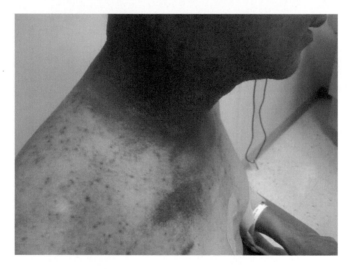

FIGURE 13.14   Patient with head and neck cancer treated with radiation. He developed erythematous plaques within the treatment field after starting epidermal growth factor receptor inhibitor.

Lymphedema has also been shown to have an increased incidence in breast cancer patients treated with adjuvant radiotherapy (30). In contrast to edema of the irradiated breast, the upper extremity is more often affected and it may occur as a consequence blockage of lymphatic vessels due to RIF.

Radiation-Induced Morphea

A rare late-stage reaction, radiation-induced morphea (RIM), has an estimated incidence of 0.2% and latency between 1 and 12 months in breast cancer patients treated with ionizing radiation (31,32). Unlike radiation-induced fibrosis, RIM has a strong immune component that follows a two-stage sequence (Figure 13.16). The first stage is the "inflammatory stage" characterized clinically by erythematous and edematous plaques. The second stage is the "burn out stage" characterized by induration, violaceous discoloration, and pain (32). There is no consensus on proper management of this rare disorder, but standard therapy for plaque morphea has been suggested (32).

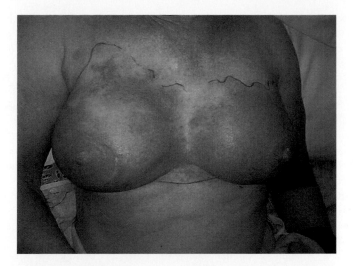

FIGURE 13.15 Edema and mastitis. Patient with breast cancer treated with skin-sparing mastectomy and radiation. She developed painful erythematous, edematous plaques on her bilateral breasts.

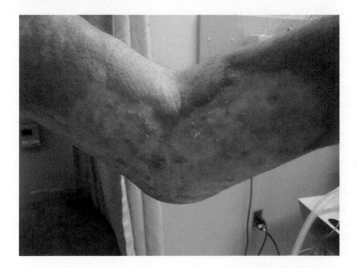

FIGURE 13.16 Patient with cutaneous B-cell lymphoma and pathologic fracture treated with radiation. He developed a progressive sclerotic plaque with bound down features restricting his range of motion. Lesion also developed hypopigmentation and telangiectasias.

REFERENCES

1. McLean AS. Early adverse effects of radiation. *Br Med Bull* 1973;29(1):69–73.
2. Emami B et al. Tolerance of normal tissue to therapeutic irradiation. *Int J Radiat Oncol Biol Phys* 1991;21(1):109–22.
3. Gunderson LL, Tepper JE, Bogart JA. *Clinical Radiation Oncology*. Philadelphia, PA: Elsevier; 2016.
4. Abeloff MD. *Abeloff's Clinical Oncology*. Philadelphia, PA: Churchill Livingstone/Elsevier; 2014.
5. Hutchinson F. Molecular basis for action of ionizing radiations. *Science* 1961;134(3478):533–8.
6. Eriksson D, Stigbrand T. Radiation-induced cell death mechanisms. *Tumour Biol* 2010;31(4):363–72.
7. Postow MA et al. Immunologic correlates of the abscopal effect in a patient with melanoma. *N Engl J Med* 2012;366(10):925–31.
8. Hickok JT, Morrow GR, Roscoe JA, Mustian K, Okunieff P. Occurrence, severity, and longitudinal course of twelve common symptoms in 1129 consecutive patients during radiotherapy for cancer. *J Pain Symptom Manage* 2005;30(5):433–42.

9. Boxman I, Lowik C, Aarden L, Ponec M. Modulation of IL-6 production and IL-1 activity by keratinocyte-fibroblast interaction. *J Invest Dermatol* 1993;101(3):316–24.

10. Bernstein EF et al. Healing impairment of open wounds by skin irradiation. *J Dermatol Surg Oncol* 1994;20(11):757–60.

11. National Cancer Institute. Common Terminology Criteria for Adverse Events v4.0. National Insitutes of Health, 2009.

12. Salvo N et al. Prophylaxis and management of acute radiation-induced skin reactions: A systematic review of the literature. *Curr Oncol* 2010;17(4):94–112.

13. Maddocks-Jennings W, Wilkinson JM, Shillington D. Novel approaches to radiotherapy-induced skin reactions: A literature review. *Complement Ther Clin Pract* 2005;11(4):224–31.

14. Hymes SR, Strom EA, Fife C. Radiation dermatitis: Clinical presentation, pathophysiology, and treatment 2006. *J Am Acad Dermatol* 2006;54(1):28–46.

15. Archambeau JO, Pezner R, Wasserman T. Pathophysiology of irradiated skin and breast. *Int J Radiat Oncol Biol Phys* 1995;31(5):1171–85.

16. Turesson I. The progression rate of late radiation effects in normal tissue and its impact on dose-response relationships. *Radiother Oncol* 1989;15(3):217–26.

17. Van Limbergen E, Rijnders A, van der Schueren E, Lerut T, Christiaens R. Cosmetic evaluation of breast conserving treatment for mammary cancer. 2. A quantitative analysis of the influence of radiation dose, fractionation schedules and surgical treatment techniques on cosmetic results. *Radiother Oncol* 1989;16(4):253–67.

18. Johns H, Morris WJ, Joiner MC. Radiation response of murine eccrine sweat glands. *Radiother Oncol* 1995;36(1):56–64.

19. Schultze-Mosgau S et al. Transforming growth factor beta1 and beta2 (TGFbeta2/TGFbeta2) profile changes in previously irradiated free flap beds. *Head Neck* 2002;24(1):33–41.

20. Herskind C et al. Fibroblast differentiation in subcutaneous fibrosis after postmastectomy radiotherapy. *Acta Oncol* 2000;39(3):383–8.

21. Delanian S, Baillet F, Huart J, Lefaix JL, Maulard C, Housset M. Successful treatment of radiation-induced fibrosis using liposomal Cu/Zn superoxide dismutase: Clinical trial. *Radiother Oncol* 1994;32(1):12–20.

22. Delanian S, Balla-Mekias S, Lefaix JL. Striking regression of chronic radiotherapy damage in a clinical trial of combined pentoxifylline and tocopherol. *J Clin Oncol* 1999;17(10):3283–90.

23. Bourgeois JF, Gourgou S, Kramar A, Lagarde JM, Guillot B. A randomized, prospective study using the LPG technique in treating radiation-induced skin fibrosis: Clinical and profilometric analysis. *Skin Res Technol* 2008;14(1):71–6.

24. Bentzen SM, Overgaard M. Relationship between early and late normal-tissue injury after postmastectomy radiotherapy. *Radiother Oncol* 1991;20(3):159–65.

25. Lanigan SW, Joannides T. Pulsed dye laser treatment of telangiectasia after radiotherapy for carcinoma of the breast. *Br J Dermatol* 2003;148(1):77–9.

26. Camidge R, Price A. Characterizing the phenomenon of radiation recall dermatitis. *Radiother Oncol* 2001;59(3):237–45.

27. Hill A, Hanson M, Bogle MA, Duvic M. Severe radiation dermatitis is related to Staphylococcus aureus. *Am J Clin Oncol* 2004;27(4):361–3.

28. Kelemen G, Varga Z, Lazar G, Thurzo L, Kahan Z. Cosmetic outcome 1–5 years after breast conservative surgery, irradiation and systemic therapy. *Pathol Oncol Res* 2012;18(2):421–7.

29. Verbelen H, Gebruers N, Beyers T, De Monie AC, Tjalma W. Breast edema in breast cancer patients following breast-conserving surgery and radiotherapy: A systematic review. *Breast Cancer Res Treat* 2014;147(3):463–71.

30. Kissin MW, della Rovere G Q, Easton D, Westbury G. Risk of lymphoedema following the treatment of breast cancer. *Br J Surg* 1986;73(7):580–4.

31. Bleasel NR, Stapleton KM, Commens C, Ahern VA. Radiation-induced localized scleroderma in breast cancer patients. *Australas J Dermatol* 1999;40(2):99–102.

32. Spalek M, Jonska-Gmyrek J, Galecki J. Radiation-induced morphea—A literature review. *J Eur Acad Dermatol Venereol* 2015;29(2):197–202.

Index

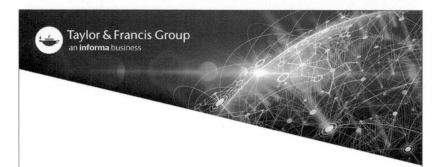